Feed the Spirit, Starve the ED

Noël Deppen

Copyright © 2022 Noël Deppen

All rights reserved. No part of this book may be reproduced or transmitted in any form or by any means, electronic or mechanical, including photocopying, recording or by any information storage and retrieval system without permission in writing from the publisher.

Hopeful Rose Publishing—Drakes Branch, VA
ISBN: 979-8-218-00768-3
Library of Congress Control Number: 2022909621
Title: *Feed the Spirit, Starve the ED*
Author: Noël Deppen
Digital distribution | 2022
Paperback | 2022

Dedication

To Lily Butler, who faithfully fought her ED as well as helping me to fight my own. Even though she lost her battle, she continues to live with me. Her encouragement and support have helped me to make it to where I am today, and for that I am forever grateful. Even though I can no longer do anything to physically help her, I can help her by helping myself and others. And that is what I intend to do.

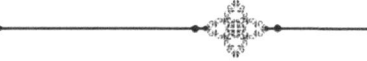

Table of Contents

Introduction vii

Chapter 1: Love 1

Chapter 2: Joy 13

Chapter 3: Peace 25

Chapter 4: Patience 36

Chapter 5: Kindness 47

Chapter 6: Goodness 56

Chapter 7 Faithfulness 64

Chapter 8: Gentleness 72

Chapter 9: Self-Control 82

Conclusion 90

Additional Helpful Tips and Tricks 92

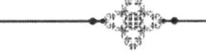

Introduction

Hi. My name is Noël Deppen, and I struggled with an eating disorder (ED) for many years. Eating disorders are devastating mental illnesses with horrible physical and psychological consequences, and I experienced a great amount of these downsides. I frequently was in and out of treatment in what often felt like a never-ending cycle. As soon as I would graduate from a program and discharge, I found myself sliding back into old harmful behaviors. The problem was that the treatment centers did not bring me the healing that I needed. They helped in terms of my physical health and with temporarily getting me back on track with normalized eating, but internally I was consumed by the same fears and thought processes. The treatment centers that I went to did provide therapy, but nothing seemed to resonate with me.

Something that people in treatment have a lot of is free time. This allowed me to devote more time to reading and studying the Bible. I even bought a journaling Bible so that I could write about how specific passages meant something to me and my recovery (this is an activity that I strongly recommend). I wanted to bring God into my recovery as much as I possibly could. While doing this, there was one passage that felt as if it was screaming at me:

Galatians 5:22-23: "But the fruit of the Spirit is love, joy, peace, patience, kindness, goodness, faithfulness, gentleness, and self-control."

Not only do I need physical food to recover from my disorder, but I also need spiritual fruit. Learning how to eat correctly and acquiring various skills are all helpful, but they are meaningless if I rely on them alone and do not turn to the Healer to heal my heart. I could feel God speaking to me on an intimate level. The answer had been there all along waiting for me to find it. This is a verse that I had read many, many times, but this was the first time that I truly realized what God wants me to hear.

I began to connect each fruit with how I can use it in recovering from the ED, and I feel as if this strengthened my recovery. I no longer was merely going through the motions; I was actually having a change of heart. The ED was no longer the one that I sought to meet my needs and wants. Instead, I learned how to seek God in every circumstance and feel whole.

To be honest, I am still working on recovery. However, each day, I dive deeper into these spiritual truths. Recovery is a process, but I know that God will be with me and with everyone else trying to overcome this disorder. Still, if you or a loved one are struggling with an eating disorder, I strongly encourage the seeking of professional treatment. Even though professional treatment by itself did not resolve my struggles, it did help significantly and provided me with the support and assistance that I, and many others, required. This book is meant as an aid and not as the sole means of assistance.

In this book, I have included various personal experiences of mine, as well as different lessons and techniques that I have learned. All Bible verses are from the English Standard Version (ESV) unless otherwise noted.

I pray that this book will help you and that through it, you will clearly hear God's message to you. Every person has their own experiences and their own unique set of techniques that are beneficial to them. I encourage you to consider what is written and incorporate whatever is beneficial to you.

This will be a difficult journey, but don't give up! You CAN conquer this disorder.

Chapter 1
Love

Love. My eating disorder was an attempt to feel loved. I wanted others to love me, but most of all, I wanted to be able to love myself.

My behaviors began because I desperately wanted to quiet the voice in my head and improve myself. I believed that if I just lost some weight, I would look better, feel more confident, and ultimately be happier. However, my small behaviors began to expand and increase. They no longer became a choice, but a compulsion. The deeper I sank into the ED, the more trapped I felt. Instead of improving my body, I began a pattern of destroying it. Instead of loving myself, I hated myself even more. I was convinced that I was worthless and unlovable.

My struggles led me on a search for truth. Since everything that I believed was being countered by professionals, I did not know what to believe. I was convinced that they were either ignorant or lying. I knew what I saw, and I knew what worked. Surely, they were the ones in the wrong! The internet was one reference that I used in my search. Obviously, one will discover many mixed messages from such source. Our world is full of diet culture that further encourages ED beliefs. Instead of receiving facts as to how I was harming myself, I was misguided to believe that I was doing the right thing.

Even though these sources may appear credible and reliable, there is only One source of truth: the Bible. It was created by the infallible God who is never wrong.

The Bible is filled with factual truths to combat the ED, as well as many promises and examples of God's love. No matter how many mistakes or faults biblical characters made, God repeatedly expressed and displayed His unconditional love. This is the love that I had desired. This is the love that is available for anyone who is willing to turn to Him.

The Bible tells us in the first chapter of the first book that we have been created by God. "So God created man in his own image, in the image of God he created him; male and female he created them" Genesis 1:27. We do not have to read far to already see how important we are. This verse is explaining how all of mankind was created in the image of God. Not just Adam, but every human being after him. This includes me and you. Every single one of us has been made in God's likeness, so this shows that we are special.

Being in the image of God does not mean that we are just like Him or that we are perfect. Rather, it displays itself through how we possess a soul, can make our own decisions, and have a sense of morality and right and wrong. No other part of creation was treasured enough to be given this gift. Only mankind can make the choice of whether they will accept Jesus Christ as their personal Savior and live in eternity with Him. It shows that we are so precious and loved by God that He has set us apart as special and desires an intimate relationship with each and every one of us. That includes me, and it includes you, too.

The chapter goes on to explain just how special we are. After each day of creation, God referred to what He had made as "good." However, after the sixth day when He created mankind, He said that we were "very good." "And God saw everything that he had made, and behold, it was very good. And there was evening and there was morning, the sixth day" Genesis 1:31. Just like being created in His likeness, this applies to every single human being that God created and will create. We are more than good enough.

The ED tries to tell us that we are not good enough and that we need to change. It points out our every flaw and whispers insecurities into our ears. We often believe what it says. However, we do not have to listen to the ED's deceptions. God has already busted those myths.

One of my core beliefs that kept me trapped in the ED was that I was not good enough. Many years of the ED screaming this lie to me caused me to believe it as truth. No matter what task I faced, I was crippled by this belief, and it impacted how I responded as well as whether I even tried. I did not want to try, because I knew that I would fail. Even if I was able to succeed, I was still convinced that certain aspects were not done well enough or that I could have and should have done better.

I attempted countless therapy techniques to try to combat this. Every assignment that my therapists would give me was tried with diligence and persistence. Unfortunately, that belief was still there.

It was firm and would not budge. Since I had believed it so deeply for so long, I required something greater. In fact, what I needed was not something, but Someone.

I have come to realize that I do not need to love myself and feel pride over my every achievement and feel apathetic towards my mistakes. I can accept that I am enough simply because God says that I am. He speaks truth, and His opinion is the only one that truly matters. I may not be able to see it yet, but until then, I will put my trust in what my Lord says.

I really enjoy the potter and clay analogy used in Isaiah 64:8: "But now, O Lord, you are our Father; we are the clay, and you are our potter; we are all the work of your hand." Like a potter sculpting clay, God shaped us the way that He wants us to be. If He had formed us and did not like how we turned out, He would have smashed the clay and started over. The fact that He did not tells us that He is pleased with how we turned out and that we are worthy of existing on this earth.

Another verse that expresses just how beautifully created we are is Psalm 139:14: "I praise you, for I am fearfully and wonderfully made. Wonderful are your works; my soul knows it very well." Since we are God's creation, this means we were wonderfully created. We are not mistakes. We are not exceptions.

I am a crocheter. One of my favorite things to crochet is teddy bears dressed in different outfits. Some of them turn out nice, while others are a bit of a struggle. Not all of them turn out exactly the way that I envision in my mind. I have my favorites that I will display and others that I abandon and store away in a bag or drawer somewhere. I used to think this was how mankind was. Some people are created good and others not so good, and I was convinced that I was one of those not-so-good creations. I was the teddy bear that was messed up and unworthy of being displayed. I was a failure, a mistake.

But God is not like man. Everything that He creates is wonderful and contains no mistakes. Each of us are woven together with precision and expertise. Even though we may feel as if we are full of flaws and mishaps, God feels differently. He created us exactly the way that He wants us to be. He is our Potter, and we are His beautiful masterpiece.

Even though the verse above compares us to clay, we are so much more than that. We are the Lord's beloved children. "See what kind of love the Father has given to us, that we should be called children of God; and so we are" 1 John 3:1. This concept can sometimes be hard for us to truly comprehend. Maybe you had a difficult relationship with your earthly father or are like me and grew up without one. My dad died when I was a baby, so I was not able to have a father during a large portion of my life. I still do not completely understand God's love, but I do know that God is the most loving Father, and He cares so much for His children. He desires good for us as we grow up, and He helps us to get there. He nourishes, provides, and raises us. He teaches us right and wrong, and He does not fail to correct us. This correction is not out of hate, but through love. He does this to prevent us from harm and to help us transform into the best version of ourselves that we can be. His love is unconditional, meaning that there is nothing you could ever do to make Him love you any less. We are enough to Him, and He loves us so much.

One thing that I really struggled with was ruminating over my flaws and mistakes. Each time I did something that I considered to be wrong or humiliating, I would be unable to get the memory out of my mind. The event would play out in my head over and over again. I would continue to relive my misery, and as a result, my opinion of myself would decline even more with each repetition. I felt as if my mistakes made me less worthy and more of a bad person. I used to wonder how God could still love me even after seeing all that was wrong with me.

But, when He looks at me, He does not see my blemishes. He sees His beloved child. Even though I emphasize my mistakes and allow them to define me as a person, He does not. Instead of viewing a creature cloaked in sin and flaws, God sees His beloved child that was washed pure and clean. He loves me for me, and He will never love me less.

Since His love is unchanging, there is also nothing that we can do to make Him love us more. I have often been misguided by the ED's claims, as well as other perfectionistic tendencies. I thought that I had to have the perfect look and the perfect body. I thought that I had to be the best at everything, from school and work to even art and games. Instead of being able to enjoy life, I was so consumed by the need to be perfect. But, I have to remind myself that that's not important to God. When we try our best, that is success to Him.

What matters is not whether we are the best, but instead God cares more about where our motives are. He values a life that is devoted to and lives for Him. This can be through showing love to others, sharing the gospel, and living life in obedience to Him and His will. That is what is beautiful: not by physical features, size, and weight, or even by talent and skill, but by our heart. "Do not let your adorning be external – the braiding of hair and the putting on of gold jewelry, or the clothing you wear – but let your adorning be the hidden person of the heart with the imperishable beauty of a gentle and quiet spirit, which in God's sight is very precious" 1 Peter 3:3-4. Also, "Charm is deceitful and beauty is vain, but a woman who fears the Lord is to be praised" Proverbs 31:30.

Changing how we look or how much we weigh is meaningless in God's eyes. If we want to make a meaningful change, it should be an internal one. Instead of changing the body, we can work to better the heart. When God sees us, that is what He sees. "But the Lord said to Samuel, 'Do not look on his appearance or on the height of his stature, because I have rejected him. For the Lord sees not as man sees: man looks on the outward appearance, but the Lord looks on the heart'" 1 Samuel 16:7.

This particular verse resonates very strongly with me. So often I found myself worrying about how I looked and how my body composition was. I devoted so much time and energy into stressing about and trying to change my body, but none of that made God's view of me change. When God looks at me, He sees my heart, and He sees that Christ dwells in me. I am His, and He is mine.

We are like His sheep, and He is our Shepherd. "What do you think? If a man has a hundred sheep, and one of them has gone astray, does he not leave the ninety-nine on the mountains and go in search of the one that went astray? And if he finds it, truly, I say to you, he rejoices over it more than over the ninety-nine that never went astray. So it is not the will of my Father who is in heaven that one of these little ones should perish" Matthew 18:12-14. Like a shepherd with his sheep, God watches over us, takes care of us, protects us, and guides us. And, like this verse states, we are so important and loved by Him that He would leave all others to bring us home to Him.

That in itself is a major expression of God's love for us, but there is more. Christ came down to earth to die for us. "For God so loved the world, that he gave his only Son, that whoever believes in him should not perish but have eternal life" John 3:16.

Mankind was sinful and separated from God, but that did not hinder God's love. He still took action then, and He does the same today. Instead of abandoning us, He waits for us and does things to draw us closer to Him. He is not bothered by our imperfections; He loves us, nonetheless. We are not loved because of what we have done, but because of who we are. None of us are horrible, unworthy, or hated, and you are NOT the exception. "Everyone needs food, but not me." "They deserve recovery, but I don't." "All people are worthy, except me." These beliefs are all pure deception. I am no less than anyone else, and neither are you. I am loved. You are loved. Everyone needs food, deserves recovery, and is oh so worthy. We are loved.

Sometimes I have struggled to accept God's love because I was so focused on other people's hate. Growing up, I had a lot of "friends" who were quick to point out my every flaw. I was always told that my hair looked hideous and my outfits were ugly. My art sucked and my performances were laughable. I was stupid and awkward, they said. Since I thought they were people that cared about me, I strongly took to heart everything they said. They were my friends! Surely I would trust their judgment. I did not feel worthy. I did not feel loved.

I have now realized that many of them were not my friends. I do not know what caused them to treat me so cruelly, but I am sure that it stems from some internal struggle that they were experiencing. It was not me; it was them. However, even though these people were not good friends, I did have one: Jesus Christ. "One who has unreliable friends soon comes to ruin, but there is a friend who sticks closer than a brother" Proverbs 18:24 (NIV). He loved me then, and He loves me now. I wish I had realized how good of a friend I had back then, but I cannot change the past. What I can change is how I respond in the future. Instead of letting others full of hate dictate my feelings and self-esteem, I choose to let that go to my loving God.

Even when others do not point out our flaws, we as human beings have the tendency to point them out for ourselves. We look at everyone else and see what they have that we do not, and this can lead to insecurities. "They look better than me." "They are better at this than me." "I wish I was deserving of love like they are." Instead of being able to acknowledge and appreciate the good we do have, we become so consumed by what we don't have or what we have that could be better.

I have had experiences where I was with a group of friends, but I was completely not present. I was trapped in my head. Instead of enjoying being with them, all I could think about was how I wished that I was more like them. All I could see were my faults, and I was convinced that since that was in the forefront of my mind, they must be thinking it, too. Instead of being happy, I allowed my mind to make me completely miserable.

The truth is that there will always be someone that seems better. However, "better" is an opinion. What one person considers to be better could be completely different from someone else, and we all value different things at different levels. Each of us are indeed different, but that is what makes us special. If everyone was the same, what would be the fun in that? We all have different areas where we shine and possess spiritual gifts. Just because one person excels in a particular area, that does not mean everyone else is less than or any less deserving of love.

And do not allow yourself to wander with the idea that you do not have an area of expertise. God has blessed all of us in many areas. They will not necessarily be the same as your family and friends, but that is what makes you unique. It may be challenging to recognize them, but it is important to practice trusting that they are there. This is something

I have had to practice, but trust me when I say that it will slowly grow with time.

I have also had to practice not dismissing compliments. Instead of assuming people compliment me to be polite or because they feel sorry for me, I can say "thank you" and trust that they mean what they say. Do not counter it or come up with a million excuses. Just acknowledge, accept, and allow your belief of the compliments to grow over time.

Compliments are not meant to make us uneasy; they are meant to acknowledge our hard work and skills and to boost our mood. When you compliment someone else, is your intention to build them up or tear them down? It will take time and practice, but if you try, you can learn to absorb the kind things that people say about you, remembering that they were spoken out of love and commemoration.

And even if you do not receive compliments from others, that's perfectly okay too. Our approval and praise absolutely do not need to come from other human beings. Their opinions are not the ones that matter. God's does. He repeatedly tells us how valued and treasured we are. Those are the compliments that are truly worthwhile.

We all are blessed in various aspects of life. We all have God-given gifts that allow us to shine and create a difference. God gave us these gifts for a reason. We cannot just abandon them because we do not feel as if we are good enough at them. Instead, we need to use them for God. "As each has received a gift, use it to serve one another, as good stewards of God's varied grace" 1 Peter 4:10. He blesses us because He loves us, and the best way for us to thank Him for His love and blessings is by using them for Him.

Since God loves us, this means that we can love ourselves. "We love because he first loved us" 1 John 4:19. I get it – it isn't easy. Honestly, I am not fully at that point myself. I am often still hyperaware and hyper-focused on my faults and flaws. I have trouble accepting them, and I also have trouble accepting that I do some things right. Until I do get to that point of self-love, I continue to focus on God's love for me, and I allow my self-love to slowly follow. I cannot rush it, but I know that it will come. As I continue to absorb God's truths and trust in His Word, I begin to inch closer and closer. I know that I can get there, and you can, too.

Chapter 2
Joy

Joy. This is often challenging for people who are struggling with eating disorders. For me, my mind was filled with so much anxiety and depression. The light of joy was either blazed by fire or clouded by fog. The little bits of joy I did experience transformed into guilt because I did not feel like I deserved to feel that way. I can clearly look back on countless moments where I could have really enjoyed myself, but instead I was miserable. It makes me sad to think of the positive memories that I was unable to obtain.

One particular memory that comes to mind is when I went on a trip to the zoo with my family. I am a strong animal lover, so this could have been a really enjoyable experience for me. Unfortunately, I allowed the ED to steal my joy. Instead of being able to appreciate my special lunch out, I was consumed by the ED's fears about the food. Throughout the meal conversation, the words spoken went in one ear and out the other. I was too busy stuck in my head calculating and criticizing the contents of what I was consuming, and thus increasing my misery.

When we began to walk around and visit the animals, I was unable to engage in the experience. I was stuck in the past ruminating over what I had just eaten. And, I was too busy paying attention to the exercise that I was doing rather than mindfully noticing my surroundings. My attention was focused inward rather than being aware of my life unfolding around me.

This could have been a very joyful time with my family, but I allowed the ED to take that from me.

That's part of what the ED is. It is a joy thief. It steals our joy and leaves us with a misguided belief that we do not deserve to feel joy unless we adhere to it and what it says. When we do not measure up to its unrealistic and unattainable expectations, it depletes us of our joy and leaves us feeling hopeless and lost.

However, God wants us to be joyful. He wants us to be able to appreciate and treasure the blessings in life that He so lovingly gives us. I know that when assessing my life and all of the good that God has given me, I have no reason to experience anything other than joy. The ED tries to put blinders on us to block us from this joy, but I have learned that instead, we can use those blinders to block out the ED. Recognize that it is trying to steal your joy and do not let it. Make a conscious decision to choose joy no matter what the ED does to try to make you feel the opposite.

One way that the ED constantly tried to steal my joy was through rigidity. The ED causes a striving for control, leading to a strong desire for order and structure and a lack of flexibility. Instead of being able to appreciate spontaneous occasions, I found myself extremely anxious and overwhelmed. Instead of going with the flow, I had to adhere to my schedule. When things were not "just right", I found myself on the edge of a nervous breakdown. I allowed myself to let this anxiety consume me rather than embracing fun and experiencing joy.

I can look back on many instances where I was given a meal that did not meet the ED's requirements. My treatment team repeatedly told me to be flexible. I can honestly say that every single session I had with my dietician, this word came up at least three times. Flexibility even became my least favorite word. "I shouldn't have to be flexible; they should just fix it and make it right!"

Over time, I eventually got the message that no matter how much I complained or petitioned, they were not going to change things. I had to learn to accept that things would not always be perfect and that I had to be flexible in order to make it through the day and progress through the treatment.

The funny thing is that the more I was flexible, the less the rigidity controlled me. Rules and requirements that would control me in the past now seem trivial and unimportant. The flexibility gave me a sense of freedom. I can live my life and face whatever comes my way without being constrained to inside the walls of my rigidity.

Rigidity is still something that from time to time shows up in my life and tries to influence me. However, now that I recognize how this only hurts instead of helping as it was intended to, I am able to take steps to conquer it. When I notice myself being held back by fears, I must make a choice as to whether I will live by fear or by faith. Fear will tell us that we will fail if we try, so we should run away to avoid getting hurt. However, faith reminds us that

God will be with us no matter what we face, and He will help us every step of the way.

Fear is such a difficult emotion to combat because it is meant to protect us. We experience fear when our minds and bodies are trying to warn us of approaching danger and keep us safe. This is all good when our fear is justified. If there is imminent danger headed our way, fear serves us well when it tells us to protect ourselves and run away. However, if our fear stems from lies and distortions, we no longer are doing ourselves a favor by listening to its warnings. Instead, we are causing ourselves to miss out. Walls may help you feel safe and secure, but if you always remain inside, you will miss out on the rest of the life that God has so graciously given. Life truly is a beautiful thing, and there is so much good in the world. Do not let the ED or rigidity or anything else prohibit you from experiencing that.

There is so much in life for us to be joyful for. Walking through nature and seeing all the beautiful plants and wildlife that exist around us is incredible. Spending time with loved ones to play a game or connect are moments to be treasured. Snuggling up with a good book or stretching out on the couch to watch television are experiences that provide comfort and relaxation. Opportunities and little blessings are moments that remind us just how blessed we truly are. And above all, feeling the presence of God with us through every moment is like being wrapped in a warm blanket of love and joy. Good exists all around us and if we acknowledge it, then there is so much wonderful joy that we are able to experience.

Not only does God want us to feel joy in times of abundance and prosperity, but also in the moments of loss and heartache. Unfortunately, even though there is much good in the world, we will inevitably encounter moments that evoke tears, pain, and heartache. During these times, experiencing joy does not come naturally. Instead, we are prone to experience anger, depression, shame, hatred, and many other emotions that cause our pain to increase. The secret to overcoming this is recognizing that we can choose what we put our attention towards. We can look at things that bring us pain, or we can turn to what brings healing. God desires for us to focus on our many blessings as opposed to the bad.

"Then our mouth was filled with laughter, and our tongue with shouts of joy; then they said among the nations, 'The Lord has done great things for them'" Psalm 126:2. There are many great things in life that God does for us. I know that for me, the fire and cloud had hidden them. But we have to look past those things. Sometimes it is harder than others, but it is always possible. When you start to recognize all the good in your life, you will see that the good truly does outweigh the bad. And, the seemingly "bad" are truly not as horrible as we think they are.

Something that I have found helpful is keeping a gratitude journal. When I started this, I would write down three things I was grateful for each day. As this became increasingly easier for me (trust me, it will get there over time), I started adding more that I would write down. As your list becomes longer and longer, you will see how there is so much beauty in each and every day. It has always been there, but we just were unable to recognize it. And, the simple act of taking time to ruminate on the good is so much more powerful and transformative that ruminating on struggles and mistakes.

If you are struggling with creating your gratitude list, try starting with small things. Maybe you had the opportunity to watch your favorite show or listen to your favorite song. Maybe you were able to get up and get ready so that you could arrive at your destination on time. Maybe a stranger smiled at you or told you "hello". Start actively looking for things to appreciate. Make every day a scavenger hunt where your goal is to find the little blessings. And know that there is a prize at the end: Joy.

If we always focus on the thorns, we will miss the roses. However, if we choose to focus on the roses, the thorns are still there, but they are not as important or scary to us. We cannot make the bad go away, but we can choose whether we will allow the bad to control us.

One "bad" that I have experienced a lot of in life is loss. Many people who were close to me have passed away due to various unfortunate circumstances. My dad, grandparents, other relatives, and friends have ceased to live throughout the years that I have resided on this earth. All of these losses were incredibly painful, but especially the loss of my dad. As I said, he died when I was a baby, but I cannot tell you how many stories of his love for me and my sisters that I have heard over the years.

Even though this was a difficult experience in my life, I have found that there are two different ways that I can interpret this. I can either allow the loss to consume me, or I can use this loss to build me up. It was very challenging, but I was able to choose joy. I choose to focus on how his presence in my life was a gain rather than how his absence is a loss.

I still miss my dad, but I know he is free from his pain. And, I still have the results of his kindness and love for me. His goodness towards me when I was young shaped me into the kind of person that I am today. Also, my dad was a special education teacher at an elementary school. Hearing all the stories of the positive impact he made on so many people's lives helped motivate me to pursue a career in which I make a meaningful impact in the lives of others. Like him, I have a passion to help others and spread love. None of this would have been possible had it not been for him.

Another loss was a dear friend of mine. In one of the treatment centers, I befriended a young girl named Lily. She was a beautiful light and was so positive and encouraging. We had many exciting and meaningful experiences together that formed a deep friendship between the two of us. She always showed how much she cared about me, and she did whatever she could to help me remain on the path of recovery.

Unfortunately, she lost her battle to her own ED and passed away. I felt devastated. I was convinced that it was my fault. I should have been a better friend. I should have been a better encourager. I also felt hopeless towards my own recovery. Since she could not do it, why would I think that I possibly could? I was discouraged, depressed, and wanted to give up.

However, I have learned to shift my perspective. Instead of feeling hopeless, I can feel hopeful. I can use her story as motivation to pursue recovery. Since I can no longer help her, what I can do is help myself. She would not want me to give up, but to keep going. She would want me to give to others what she gave to me.

I am thankful that Lily was a part of my life. She showed me so much love and kindness, and I have many memories of moments that I experienced with her that I can treasure. She helped me in so many ways, and this has helped to mold me into the individual that I am today. Even though she was young, I know that she fulfilled her purpose by showing love and helping others.

"In the day of prosperity be joyful, and in the day of adversity consider: God has made the one as well as the other" Ecclesiastes 7:14. God did not create the difficult times to torture us. God is love, and everything He does stems from this love. In fact, the seemingly negative situations actually serve a divine purpose. There is a reason for everything, and there is something that God desires for you to gain by enduring each difficult situation. "Count it all joy, my brothers, when you meet trials of various kinds, for you know that the testing of your faith produces steadfastness. And let steadfastness have its full effect, that you may be perfect and complete, lacking in nothing" James 1:2-4.

Even though these losses were incredibly difficult, I know that God had a purpose. There was a reason why God brought these individuals home when He did. Also, there was a reason why God had me experience these losses. We may not always understand, but we can trust that God knows and has a plan. And when our rough situations are especially rocky, we can find comfort when we lean on Him.

In the moment, it can be incredibly difficult to find the rose in the thorns, but we are able to see it if we look hard enough and seek God through the pain. Some of the benefits that I have gained from rougher situations are learning lessons, becoming closer to God, being an inspiration to others, and being able to recognize the blessings that I do have. Sometimes the deliverance from torrential waves to peaceful waters also helps us to better appreciate the good. "When I thought, 'My foot slips,' your steadfast love, O Lord, held me up. When the cares of my heart are many, your consolations cheer my soul" Psalm 94:18-19.

One example where I experienced all of this was when I was in treatment. The lesson that I learned was the consequences of my actions. Listening to the ED took me away from home and school, ended me up in treatment centers, caused physical complications, fractured relationships, and did not even bring me the relief that I was seeking. I also realized the blessings that I already had. I have a wonderfully supportive family and so many other things going for me out in the real world, not to mention an amazing God who will forever be with me. Treatment also brought me closer to God. I had much more time to dive into God's Word and pray, and it reminded me even more about how much I need him. And, the joy that I felt coming home from a long treatment stay is inexpressible.

I also humbly admit that I have been able to be an inspiration to others in treatment. As far as meals, seeing me push past my thoughts and fears helped others to do the same. Being able to share what works for me has taught others new tips and tricks. Seeing me reading my Bible has even motivated others to dive deeper into their faith, and it has opened opportunities for me to share the hope that I have with others. None of this would have been possible had it not been for the trials that I endured.

Often in the midst of these trials, it is hard to see the light up ahead. However, I have found that sometimes you do not need to look forward; looking backwards can help, too. God has done many good things for us in the past that can give us hope for the future.

Looking back can remind ourselves of how God has brought us out of trials in the past, which can revitalize our hope that God will get us through this current trial. For example, some meals that I would be faced with caused me to feel extreme fear. I was convinced that I would be unable to complete them. However, when I looked back, I could remember various other meals that also seemed impossible yet were not. Since God got me through all of those challenging meals in the past, He can get me through this one, too.

It is so comforting to know that these great things are not only in the past. "Oh give thanks to the Lord, for he is good; for his steadfast love endures forever" 1 Chronicles 16:34. Since God's love is forever, His good is forever. I know that much good is to come. God promises to make everything work out not just for good, but for my good and for your good. "And we know that for those who love God all things work together for good, for those who are called according to his purpose" Romans 8:28.

God is in control. I do not know what is going on behind the scenes, but He does. Even though things may seem hopeless and like a tangled-up mess, I know that God is already in the process of weaving together a beautiful masterpiece.

Your life may seem like a mess right now. It may feel as if you are experiencing trial after trial after trial. You may be consumed by a traumatic event that occurred in the past and are struggling to move forward. You may be stuck in a situation right now in which it feels as if there is no way out. Just know that it's okay to cry. It's okay to not understand. It's okay to feel whatever emotion you feel. The important thing is that even through it all, you turn to God. Cry out to Him. Turn to the Lord in prayer and ask for His comfort and His joy. And hang onto the hope that everything will be okay. Only God can provide us with the strength to move through our darkest moments. Only God can provide us with the ability to feel joy in the midst of heartache.

The events of our past do not define us. Things that people said and did to us are not our fault and are not things that have to be carried with us into the future. Our current experiences will not go on forever, and we do not have to allow them to hold us back. "Weeping may tarry for the night, but joy comes with the morning" Psalm 30:5. Just as night turns to day, so do trials turn to victories. And nights can bring joy, too, when we recognize the moon and the stars that bring light and peace.

We cannot always control what is thrown our way, but we can control how we respond. Joy is a choice. With God, we can choose joy even in the worst circumstances. "Rejoice in the Lord always; again I will say, rejoice" Philippians 4:4.

Now I make positive memories. I put away my negative feelings and fears, and instead I choose joy. It isn't easy, and I often fall short. I still have many instances where I allow depression to temporarily overwhelm me and for anxieties to hold me back. But, the more I practice and continue to try, the better I am at it. I never thought that I would feel this way, but I do. The same is true for you. You can experience joy again. Remember that the greatest things in life are those you work for. It may be hard, and it will take time, but with God, you've got this!

Chapter 3
Peace

Peace. I can honestly tell you that the ED has brought me absolutely no peace, although it continually promised to. "Just look a certain way and you will be at peace with your body." "Just don't eat that and everything will be much better." "Just engage in this behavior and all of those painful feelings will go away." Unfortunately, they never did go away. I may have felt periods of temporarily relief, but these were just that: temporary. Over the long-term, engaging in the ED just made my anxiety and distress even worse.

I have learned the "peace" that the ED promised to provide was not what my soul desires. Rather, that peace can only be found in Jesus Christ. "Peace I leave with you; my peace I give to you. Not as the world gives do I give to you. Let not your hearts be troubled, neither let them be afraid" John 14:27.

When we turn to Jesus, He gives us true comfort. He promises to be with us and provide for our needs. He walks with us and wipes away our tears and bandages our wounds. He carries our burdens and takes away worries that are unnecessary. The ED, on the other hand, adds worries.

The ED tried to tell me that I needed to worry about what I ate and about what I looked like, but

God tells us that we do not need to worry about these things. "Therefore I tell you, do not be anxious about your life, what you will eat or what you will drink, nor about your body, what you will put on. Is not life more than food, and the body more than clothing?" Matthew 6:25.

I have found this verse to be incredibly meaningful to my recovery. Meals do not need to be a source of anxiety for me, and neither does my body. I do not need to stress over the calories or other nutritional content of my meal. I do not need to be fixated on whether or not it was prepared according to the ED's rules and standards. I do not need to eat my meal a certain way or adhere to a set of strict rituals. I do not need to earn my food or compensate after eating. And I do not need to stress over my body either. Fat on my body is not disgusting; it is protecting my body and my organs. Scars, wrinkles, acne, and other blemishes do not make me flawed; they make me unique. These "faults" show that I am a human being who has lived life. I have experienced pain, but I have also experienced joy. I am a unique and special individual, and so are you.

I also really resonate with the last part. There is so much more to life than food. In the depths of the ED, food was always on my mind. I was always either thinking about what I just ate, what I was currently eating (or not eating), or about what I was going to eat in the future. I thought about how to burn off or eliminate what I had eaten, and I thought about what I needed to do to ease my food anxiety. But, food does not need to be the focus of my life. There are people and activities and so many other things that are far more beneficial, and much more enjoyable, to devote my attention to. Food is something that is definitely worth focusing on if it is a positive experience for you, but if your preoccupation is just causing you more distress and pain, then it is not beneficial to worry about. The same is true for our bodies. Body love is good, but body hate and criticism are essentially abuse.

Also, there is so much more to my body than how I look. My body allows me to do so many wonderful things, and that is what matters.

My body allows me to hug my mom. It lets me play and cuddle with my cats. It enables me to walk through nature and enjoy the beautiful sights and sounds that God has blessed me with the opportunity to experience. It allows me to participate in mindful movement, where I move my body in a way that feels good and brings me joy. During these moments, I find that my body shape and the number on the scale are insignificant. Life is not about how my body is, but what it does, and my body allows me to make connections and have fun.

Not only are our bodies exactly the way they need to be, but everything is. God knows everything, and He knows exactly what is needed when. We can have peace in knowing that God is in control.

When I think about this, I think about my times trying to get into treatment centers. Each time I tried to go, there was always something that got in my way, whether it was my health or insurance or a global pandemic. However, I now know that this was God's way of making the timing work out. The people who I was able to interact with would not have been the same, and God knew that both me and them could benefit from being together. The delays also prepared me to be in the proper headspace and have a greater desire and motivation to recover. And, all of my treatment stays led up to the final one. In each, I developed skills and insight that I would not have developed had I not gone. Therefore, even though the waiting and being in treatment numerous times was incredibly painful, I know that it was God, who knows all, working things out for my good.

God is more than just omniscient (all-knowing); He is also omnipotent (all-powerful). He is stronger than anything we could possibly encounter. "When I am afraid, I put my trust in you. In God, whose word I praise, in God I trust; I shall not be afraid. What can flesh do to me?" Psalm 56:3-4. We do not need to fear anything, because we know Who is on our side. God is with us, and He will protect us from anything that rises against us. Whether you are fearful during a challenging meal or are in a situation where you need to seek treatment, you can rest assured in knowing that God is with you and will protect you. Food will not hurt you. Through treatment, you will not be alone. In these experiences, as well as whatever trial you face, our all-powerful God will be with you.

Instead of resorting to fear and panic, we have the awesome gift of God's provision, and we can trust in Him. Two Bible verses that speak on this are Joshua 1:9: "Have I not commanded you? Be strong and courageous. Do not be frightened, and do not be dismayed, for the Lord your God is with you wherever you go" and Isaiah 41:10: "Fear not, for I am with you; be not dismayed, for I am your God; I will strengthen you, I will help you, I will uphold you with my righteous right hand."

With God on our side, we not only do not have to fear, but we can stand tall, bold, and confident. Confidence does not come from feeling like we look good enough or belief that we are competent enough. Instead, our confidence comes from knowing Who we have with us.

With that being said, our human nature will still cause us to fear. It is in these times that we can turn to God to ease our worries and provide us with the strength to stand. Instead of giving in the fear, we must give over our fears to God.

Whenever I realize that fear is rising within me, I take a deep breath, remind myself of these verses on courage, and say a small prayer, "God, give me the strength to get through this, and please help everything to be okay." Not only are you asking God for help, but this also serves as a reminder to yourself that God is with you. The more you say this and other prayers, the more your connection with God will grow and your faith that He will be with you will expand. Sometimes the smallest prayers can be the most heartfelt and make the most significant impact.

A time that I had to frequently say this prayer, and still often do, is mealtimes. The ED twists reality and tries to claim that food is meant to be feared. However, this lie could not be further from the truth! A question in 1 Corinthians 9:4 asks, "Do we not have the right to eat and drink?" We do! As human beings, we both need and deserve food. Food is a blessing meant for enjoyment. The Bible truly does have verses for every situation, and that even includes how eating is a good thing. Ecclesiastes has three important verses that touch on this:

"There is nothing better for a person than that he should eat and drink and find enjoyment in his toil. This also, I saw, is from the hand of God" Ecclesiastes 2:24

"And I commend joy, for man has nothing better under the sun but to eat and drink and be joyful, for this will go with him in his toil through the days of his life that God has given him under the sun" Ecclesiastes 8:15

"Go, eat your bread with joy, and drink your wine with a merry heart, for God has already approved what you do" Ecclesiastes 9:7

As you can see, God wants us to eat food and enjoy it. He wants us to be able to have cake on our birthday and candy during holidays. He wants us to enjoy pizza night with our family and go out to eat with friends. These were all things that in the depths of the ED, I was unable to do. But, I am realizing that these are experiences meant to be treasured, not dreaded. These are special moments that we can look forward to with excitement and look back on with a smile.

Food was never meant to cause anxiety or guilt. Food is not bad, and it is not something that makes us bad. The Bible tells us that we cannot be made unclean by the food that we eat. "And he said to them, 'Then are you also without understanding? Do you not see that whatever goes into a person from outside cannot defile him, since it enters not his heart but his stomach, and is expelled?' (Thus he declared all foods clean)" Mark 7:18-19.

During the rough times with the ED, I had what I called "good foods" and "bad foods" which categorized foods based on how safe or unsafe the ED convinced me that they were. However, God does not believe in this separation. God created all food and has called all good and clean. Food does not defile us. "It is not what goes into the mouth that defiles a person, but what comes out of the mouth; this defiles a person" Matthew 15:11.

Changing how we eat does not improve us or make us better individuals, just as eating a certain way does not make us bad. Living life in wickedness and sin is what destroys us, not what we eat.

Engaging in unhealthy relations with food actually does the opposite of bettering us; it is harmful. Food is a necessity, and every human being requires it to live. "Now I urge you to take some food. You need it to survive" Acts 27:34 (NIV). It equips us to carry out tasks and to fulfill God's will. When I was deep in the ED, I had neither the physical nor the mental strength to do anything, thus prohibiting me from fulfilling my purpose. However, adequate nutrition allows me to function and fully live!

It allows me to engage with others in various activities, conversations, and play. It lets me go to college and complete tasks. My sleep is even better now because of the nutrition that I am allowing my body to receive. I have the strength now that I did not have before, and I have the mental energy to think and process and experience all that life has to offer. Altering food intake may adjust your weight, but it will also negatively affect so many other aspects of your life, and these losses are definitely not worth it.

Not only does food help with one's physical and mental wellbeing, but it also helps with emotion regulation. Many times, I have cried over tiny things, been extremely anxious about nothing, or lashed out when I should not have all because my body was in starvation mode. During times where I was really struggling with the ED, I acted in ways that I deeply regret. I became a completely different person, and this change was not for the better. Letting the ED drive the car can hinder the godly qualities the Lord desires for His children to express. I personally want to be as Christ-like as I can possibly be and to never be that version of myself ever again. Simply changing the level of nourishment that I received made a significant difference.

Another area in which we can have peace is by focusing on the Lord's promise of meeting our every need. "And my God will supply every need of yours according to his riches in glory in Christ Jesus" Philippians 4:19. An important fact to remember regarding this is that God knows our needs better than we do. I have often felt as if my needs were not being met and wondered why God was not fulfilling His promise. However, He was, is, and always will. We simply must trust that He knows what we need even when we do not.

We do not need to stress over not having worldly things because we know that our needs are met. I may not have the smartest brain, but I am still able to think and learn and process information. I may not be the best at art, but I am still able to find enjoyment through it and express myself. I may not have the thinnest body, but it enables me to live my life and serve the Lord.

This body acceptance piece is very difficult and is something that I am personally still working on. I do not know if I will ever reach body-love, but I do not need to. Instead, I can accept that this is the body that God gave me, and it does what I need it to do. I may not like it, but I can accept it. And, I know that one day when I go home to be with the Lord, I will be given a new body. 2 Corinthians 5:1-5 (GNT) says, "For we know that when this tent we live in—our body here on earth—is torn down, God will have a house in heaven for us to live in, a home he himself has made, which will last for ever. And now we sigh, so great is our desire that our home which comes from heaven should be put on over us; by being clothed with it we shall not be without a body. While we live in this earthly tent, we groan with a feeling of oppression; it is not that we want to get rid of our earthly body, but that we want to have the heavenly one put on over us, so that what is mortal will be transformed by life. God is the one who has prepared us for this change, and he gave us his Spirit as the guarantee of all that he has in store for us."

It is true that these earthly bodies are not perfect. There are blemishes and blotches. There are things that our bodies struggle to do. However, we can still appreciate our bodies for how they are. God created us this way because we are beautiful to Him. And our bodies have the capacity to live life and experience all that it has to offer. Even individuals with various disabilities are still loved and beautiful to God, and they still can embrace life. Disabilities and limitations do not make us any less than; they just mean that we must approach life differently. Everyone is different and unique in their own way. None of us can do everything perfectly. Instead, we can all do things our own special way. And that's just another factor in what makes us unique.

We do not need to loathe our bodies because of what they have that is wrong or what they do not have. Instead, we can accept where we are right now and know that one day, our bodies will be made new.

We can find peace in God's promises, because they will come true. "Sovereign Lord, you are God! Your covenant is trustworthy, and you have promised these good things to your servant" 2 Samuel 7:28 (NIV). There is much good that God has promised for us. I encourage you to explore God's many promises in your own personal Bible study time. Take time to see how they connect with you, and especially with your recovery. Write down the ones that resonate with you most and remind yourself of these promises often. They will fill you with peace and provide you with the hope to keep going despite what the ED tries to throw your way. The ED wants to disrupt your peace and cause you to anxiously run back to it, but do not let it!

Peace is one of the keys to freedom from the ED. Thankfully, Jesus Christ has promised to be our peace. Seek Him instead of the ED, and your life will drastically change. With God, you can find true peace.

The Lord has been with you in the past, He is with you now, and He will continue to be with you. You will always have the presence of the Comforter, and you never have to fear the storms that blow your way. He will equip you, strengthen you, and love you through it all. In this, we can experience peace.

Chapter 4
Patience

Patience. As a very anxious person, I tend to struggle a lot with patience. I have frequently been called impatient, and as much as I'd like to deny it, I know that it is true. I struggle with needing everything to happen right away so that I know it will be okay and so that I do not have time to ruminate over all the possible catastrophic outcomes. If I did not receive an important email or grade quick enough, I convinced myself that I had forgotten to send or turn something in. If people did not move quick enough, I feared that we would be late, and that tardiness would be accompanied by detrimental consequences. If someone did not immediately respond, I feared that they had died. If an event did not happen right away, I would come up in my mind with how the entire event would occur from beginning to end with everything going completely awry. My brain was convinced that tragedy was going to occur, and the delays of life seemed to reinforce this fear.

However, even though this impatience stems from a place of concern and care, it is in no way beneficial. It is neither productive nor positive. It only causes me to be more anxious and miserable. And, it is often difficult for the people with whom we are being impatient towards. All in all, it is a lose-lose situation.

Thankfully, there are many truths in God's Word that show us why patience is the way to go as well as providing us with encouragement to help us develop this ability to wait. First off, the Bible tells us that the Lord's timing is perfect. Since He knows all- past, present, and future- He knows what is best, way better than we do. "But do not overlook this one fact, beloved, that with the Lord one day is as a thousand years, and a thousand years as one day. The Lord is not slow to fulfill his promise as some count slowness, but is patient toward you, not wishing that any should perish, but that all should reach repentance" 2 Peter 3:8-9.

We may feel as if something is taking too long to occur, but in reality, everything is working out at the right timing according to God's plan. It may feel slow, but it is actually moving right on schedule. It most likely will not be according to our timetable, but just know that God knows more than we do. His timing is far superior to anything we could ever come up with.

And, His plan is for good. "The Lord is good to those who wait for him, to the soul who seeks him. It is good that one should wait quietly for the salvation of the Lord" Lamentations 3:25-26. Instead of stressing during the wait, we are to trust that the Lord will give us what we need when we need it. Only when we wait for His goodness are we able to experience the amazing blessings that He has planned for us. Only then are we able to be strengthened and renewed. "But they who wait for the Lord shall renew their strength; they shall mount up with wings like eagles; they shall run and not be weary; they shall walk and not faint" Isaiah 40:31.

Patience is actually a very important part of ED recovery. As unfortunate as it is, recovery is not a quick and easy process. It takes a lot of time and determination. The first time we try to fly, we may fall flat on our face. And that's okay. The important thing is that we keep trying. Don't let your struggles prevent you from continuing to try. Instead, use what you have learned from your past experiences to influence what methods you attempt in the future. If taking a leap is too much, it may be more beneficial to take small steps. Even though you will not reach your destination right away, these steps will best prepare and equip you to successfully overcome the challenges that come your way.

I personally had to take these small steps when overcoming my fear foods. Instead of starting with the foods that I was most scared of, I worked my way up. I needed to develop mastery and confidence. So, I began by attempting my lowest tier fears. I set realistic goals: not too easy, but not too overwhelming. As I overcame the easier battles, I was able to continue climbing up the ladder. It's a process. Even though I did not get to the top right away, I was being continually renewed and strengthened.

Like advancing up the fear food pyramid, our whole lives are a series of growth and improvement. Even though we are not perfect now, God is not finished with us yet. He has amazing things planned for each and every one of us. "For I know the plans I have for you, declares the Lord, plans for welfare and not for evil, to give you a future and a hope" Jeremiah 29:11. And, that future is oh so beautiful. "He has made everything beautiful in its time" Ecclesiastes 3:11.

Jeremiah 29:11 is a verse that has really helped me be willing to pursue recovery. I used to think that my life was meaningless and that I would suffer with the ED forever. What's the point of going to treatment if my efforts were doomed to fail? The ED just seemed so loud and so controlling, and I feared that I would never overcome it. Especially since I had repeatedly attempted recovery but continued to relapse, my hope was nearly depleted, and I was convinced that my life was destined for failure.

However, our efforts are not doomed to fail. God does not set His children up for failure, but for success. I, and you too, have a future ahead of us that is beautiful and prosperous. It may not be exactly the way we imagine or desire for it to go, but it will be according to God's glory.

All growing up, I had planned out how my future would play out. I knew all the academic achievements that I would receive, both in grade school and in college, and was sure of my future career. I would win this then and achieve this by such and such time. I had created my checklist and all I had to do was advance through the list.

Unfortunately, the ED and treatment completely disrupted my checklist of accomplishments, causing me to take a different path in life. I felt like a failure. As the rest of the people my age were moving along in life, I seemed to be stunted and not progressing. My high school and college were moved to online, and I frequently had to take academic breaks for treatment. The life that I once knew and what I had expected to come was completely out the window.

This is still something that is hard for me to accept. I want to be further along in college by now. I want to be further along in adulting. However, God has a different plan for me. I will get there, but it will just take a little more time. And that is okay. I am no less than compared to anyone else. I am not a failure, or a disappointment, or any other cruel name that I or anyone else can come up with. God knows that this route is the most beneficial for me. I do not understand it, but thankfully He does.

And, through taking these academic breaks, I have received some benefits. I have learned to have a greater appreciation for my education opportunities instead of taking them for granted. Plus, through treatment, I have learned various skills and techniques that I would not have acquired elsewhere. I have made connections with people who I otherwise would never have met, and I have had experiences that grew who I am as a person. Most of all, these breaks saved my life so that I can continue with school and pursue the career that God has designed for me to do.

Our efforts are not in vain. At the top of the mountain, there is a wonderful future waiting for us. The climb may be long and hard, but no mountain goes on forever; there is always a peak.

When it feels as if you will never reach the top, do not lose faith in the Lord and turn to other means of meeting your needs such as the ED. Sometimes when my anxiety and depression were overwhelming, I would turn to the ED. Instead of waiting for God to soothe me with His peace and love, I would turn to the ED in an attempt to fill my cup.

It may not feel like it, but the ED is an idol. It is something that is stealing your worship away from God. And, the Bible clearly states that one cannot divide their worship. "No one can serve two masters, for either he will hate the one and love the other, or he will be devoted to the one and despise the other" Matthew 6:24. As much as we feel like giving in to the ED is innocent, it actually is drawing us further and further away from the Lord. This path seems okay, but it really is the exact opposite. "There is a way that seems right to a man, but its end is the way to death" Proverbs 14:12.

The ED is very conniving and deceiving. When I would listen to it, I fully thought that I was doing the right thing. I thought that I was taking care of my body and was helping to better it. I thought that I was giving myself what I wanted and needed. In reality, it was bringing me pain and suffering, and many times it brought me to the doorstep of death.

"The thief comes only to steal and kill and destroy. I [Jesus] came that they may have life and have it abundantly" John 10:10. I was rescued by the One who gives abundant life when I realized that He is the One I need. He is the One I am to follow. The ED brings destruction, but Jesus brings life and healing.

That being said, we will still encounter painful times. The important factor is how we respond. Instead of resorting to the ED during times of suffering, we can look at these times with a positive perspective. "Not only that, but we rejoice in our sufferings, knowing that suffering produces endurance, and endurance produces character, and character produces hope" Romans 5:3-4.

This verse connects very much to what we referred to in treatment as "urge surfing". Whenever we had the urge to engage in a destructive behavior, such as purging or self-harm, we were taught to "ride the wave". This involves sitting with the uncomfortable urge and waiting for it to past. To be honest, it feels like suffering. Sitting and not acting on what feels like an uncontrollable impulse is in no way simple or pleasant. To help us get through, we were taught to make commitments: "I will wait x minutes and then reevaluate my urge." In order to help ease the discomfort during the waiting, it is helpful to distract ourselves. Do something that moves the urge away from the forefront of your mind. The thought will still be there, but it will not be the sole thought that you are consumed by. After x minutes, we reassess. "I could do x minutes, so maybe I can wait x more." You will be amazed by how long you are able to hold out. After time continues to go by, the urge will fade away, and you will have achieved a victory over the ED.

Sometimes through this process, you will give in. This does not mean that you have failed. You tried, and every effort is increasing your strength and endurance. As you continue to practice, you will become stronger and stronger. The urge will disappear after an increasingly shorter amount of time. You will grow in your recovery and will have more power against the ED. And, hope of full recovery will start to blossom.

When we endure struggles and come out victorious, we become stronger. Even though I do not enjoy sitting through the difficult times, I have found that my hope is enough to get me through. I know that my God is good and will deliver me, and this reminder helps the rough times seem less rocky.

Hope is what got me through my times in treatment. Being in a hospital 24/7 and constantly being exposed to the things I feared most was in no way an enjoyable experience. All I wanted to do was give up and leave against medical advice (AMA). I did AMA a few times. I allowed the ED to overwhelm me. However, this does not mean that I failed. I just lost a battle. Thankfully, I was able to recognize that I truly needed treatment, so I returned.

The urge to AMA inevitably arose again, but I worked to resist it. Recovery was going to be hard, but I could not just run from my fears. I had to fight. As I continued to persist despite my struggles, I realized that maybe I could do this. Maybe I could eat this way and be okay. Also, as I continued to nourish myself, I started to rediscover my true character. I started to return, while the ED slowly began to fade away. The returning of myself brought hope. Maybe I can recover. Maybe I can have a life outside of the ED. Maybe.

Another thing I struggled with was comparisons. In treatment, I was able to observe many different people progressing at vastly different rates. The last time that I was in treatment, my progression was incredibly slow. I was not able to meet goals or move up in levels as quickly as I wanted to. I compared myself to others and even to myself during previous treatment stays. I felt unsuccessful. I felt weak. I felt like a failure.

My treatment team would always remind me that this was my own pace and was best for me. Instead of breezing through the program and not really addressing the issues, I was actively working through my problems at the speed that I needed. Rather than shutting down and mindlessly "doing the things", I was constantly fighting the battle in my head. Sometimes I would lose a battle and be unable to complete a meal, but at least I was fighting. The more I fought, the more stamina and strength I built. Soon, fear foods became allies instead of enemies.

So, do not beat yourself up over not progressing as quickly as you would like to in recovery. Even if your journey is long and contains many ups and downs, that is completely okay. As long as you keep fighting and turning to God for your strength, that is the absolute best that one could possibly do.

I also would like to add that you do not need to beat yourself up over being on the other end of the spectrum. Having a speedy recovery makes your ED no less valid. Like I said, God's timing is perfect. He has everyone experience whatever they experience for the time that is best for them.

Wherever you are in your recovery journey, or any life journey, turning to God through prayer is a great comfort. "Rejoice in hope, be patient in tribulation, be constant in prayer" Romans 12:12. This verse has become my personal motto. Even though I face many difficult battles, I know I must stick them out and patiently wait until the end. Throughout the difficult times, and even in the better moments, I have learned to continue to pray and stay connected to God. And, I always keep my goals in mind and hang on to my hope for recovery. "But as for me, I will look to the Lord; I will wait for the God of my salvation; my God will hear me" Micah 7:7.

The more you turn to God and your values and your goals, the less likely you are to resort to the ED. It will still try to sneak in, and it oftentimes will for a bit, but you will have more secret weapons to combat it. Never lose sight of what is important to you.

For anyone pursuing recovery, I just want to warn you that it is a long, difficult process. There are many twists and turns, hills and valleys, but the end result is all worth it. And, you CAN get there. Like I said, I have had to go to numerous treatment centers and have experienced many relapses before it finally stuck. But each time, I was not alone. The Lord was continuing to be with me and strengthen me each and every day, and He will be with you, as well.

The Lord DOES help His children, and He DOES strengthen them. "He gives strength to the weary and increases the power of the weak" Isaiah 40:29 (NIV). This is just one of God's many promises. He also promises to restore His people. "And after you have suffered a little while, the God of all grace, who has called you to his eternal glory in Christ, will himself restore, confirm, strengthen, and establish you" 1 Peter 5:10. Not only that, but He promises to be with us during the waiting. "Be strong and courageous. Do not fear or be in dread of them, for it is the Lord your God who goes with you. He will not leave you or forsake you" Deuteronomy 31:6.

Like I said, recovery is a process, and I am not even fully there yet. But, I know that as I continue to walk this path, God will be right there along with me, and He will help me to experience full recovery. The same is true for you. You are not in this alone. You have a constant companion with you, and He will help you through the waiting. Just keep close to God, and don't give up!

Chapter 5
Kindness

Kindness. This is a more difficult subject to touch on because it can often lead people to feel guilty and as if they are a bad person. I know that I have often felt this way. However, that is not at all what this chapter is meant to do. Rather than focusing on what you are not doing, this chapter is designed to motivate and encourage what you can do.

What I mean by kindness is thinking about others in relation to your recovery. Even though the ED is very harmful to you, it can also hurt those around you. Thus, choosing recovery helps you as well as others. "Let each of you look not only to his own interests, but also to the interests of others" Philippians 2:4.

That being said, choosing to remain in your ED is an act that is not rooted in kindness. It affects those around you in negative ways, even though that is not your intention. The ED works so that all you can see and focus on is itself, which can prohibit you from being aware of or working to change the consequences that it can have on other people. Just as the ED causes you pain, this pain can spread onto others whom you care about.

One situation that I vividly remember in which I was not focusing on kindness occurred during the first year that I really struggled with the ED. My intake was dwindling increasingly, and my family had become well aware and highly concerned. One day when I portioned a miniscule amount for my breakfast, my sister made an attempt to motivate me to eat more. She told me that she would eat the same thing as I did. I did not want her to starve herself, but I was so scared and was unable to get myself to eat more. I was not letting kindness rule my actions; I was being consumed by the ED.

Not only did the ED hurt the people who I was in a relationship with, but it also fractured some relationships. That sister and I were always very close. However, when the ED became stronger and I began to increasingly act on additional behaviors, it upset her, causing her to distance herself from me. The last thing I wanted to do was hurt her or lose her, but that is exactly what happened.

"For if your brother is grieved by what you eat, you are no longer walking in love. By what you eat, do not destroy the one for whom Christ died" Romans 14:15. When I realized how much my eating habits affected her and our relationship, I realized that I needed to make a change. Still, even after I had the desire to change, it took a lot of hard work and effort. I often fell short and gave in to the ED. This is not because I did not care, but rather because eating disorders are very cruel and difficult illnesses. Even though I continued to sometimes struggle, I was still fighting with her in mind, and through that, I was working to live in kindness.

As an aside, I would just like to emphasize that there is a major difference between trying and struggling versus not trying at all. When someone is putting in motivation and effort, they are living in kindness. No one is perfect, so one cannot expect recovery to be a perfect and easy journey. I think that this concept is very important for support people to understand. It is impossible for someone who has not lived with an ED to know what it is like. EDs are often extremely misunderstood. EDs are not a choice. We choose whether we fight it, but even if we choose to, that does not mean we will win 100% of the time.

And for those of you who are struggling, you know your heart. Do not allow anyone to put you down when you know how hard you are trying. Even when you fall short, every effort is a huge victory. Just know that even if no one else can see your fight, God can, and He is incredibly proud of you for fighting the good fight. And know that I am so proud of you, too.

Many years I experienced an immense amount of guilt over all that I put my sister through, and much of that guilt lingers with me today. However, rather than looking at the past, I choose to look towards the future. I now use these incidences as motivators to make wise and caring decisions. I may have made harmful choices in the past, but God has forgiven me, and He will be with me as I make choices in the future. I will turn to Him to help me live in love and kindness, and I will not allow the ED to hurt my loved ones anymore.

My sister and I are rebuilding our relationship. To be honest, we are not as close as we were before. However, our bond is growing, and I am sure that it will blossom into something so beautiful and unimaginable. Also, through the loss, I now have a greater appreciation for the relationship that I have with her. It is amazing how much we take for granted and how much our lives are changed when we lose things. I love both of my sisters so much, and I am committed to living in kindness to never allow anything to happen to lose any of them ever again.

As much as I would love to say that these were all the ways that the ED has hurt those close to me, unfortunately this is not the case. It often caused my emotions to blow up and overflow onto my loved ones in a not so loving way. Many times when my mom would try to counter the ED, I would lash out at her. I did not want her telling me what to do differently, I did not want her to tell me what I was doing wrong, and I did not want her to say anything that was against the ED. These outbursts were not me though; they were from the ED. However, I was the one allowing it to take the reins. I felt weak and as if I could not fight back.

But with God, we can. We can follow the command found in Ephesians 4:29: "Let no corrupting talk come out of your mouths, but only such as is good for building up, as fits the occasion, that it may give grace to those who hear." Even when the ED is trying to dictate what we say, we can instead turn to God. We can let the Holy Spirit guide the words that we speak instead of allowing the ED to lead us into corruption.

This can be very difficult sometimes. When all we see is what the ED is telling us, we are more prone to act impulsively based on what it wants us to do. What I have found to be helpful is to do a lot of reflection. After I had calmed down from a confrontational interaction, I would honestly ask myself why this happened. Why did I act the way that I did, and why did the other person respond in the way that they responded? The ED would tell me that I did nothing wrong and that I was in the right. However, if I truly was honest with myself, I would recognize that yes, I was stressed, but I should not have acted the way I did. And, even if my emotional response was justified, it was not the best way for me to respond. Then, I would apologize to the other person and make amends to the best of my ability. We cannot always make up for our mistakes, but oftentimes we can, and it is definitely worth trying. The more I reflected on my interactions, the more I became increasingly aware of when I would allow my anxieties and fears to control me, thus helping me to put a stop to it before things escalated. I am not perfect, but my actions are becoming much more grounded in kindness.

In addition to speaking out when I should not have, I have also shut out and stopped speaking to important people in my life. The ED works to eliminate everyone from your life except itself. It bombards you with depression, insecurities, and isolative behaviors that take you away from the people who matter most. Instead of living life in the "real world" and interacting with those we love, it works to keep us trapped in our heads, and the only voice that we can interact with is itself.

The best way to combat this is by engaging in opposite action. Do the opposite of what the ED wants you to do. Recognize what is important to you and let that be the map to guide you rather than obeying the ED. If recovery and connections are important to you, put yourself out there! Instead of running away from people, you can approach them. Let yourself express the love in your heart and allow yourself to fully feel the love of others.

Because of the ED, I have sadly lost so many valued friends. Due to my fears and the isolation the ED caused me to have, I just could not get myself to keep up with the relationships. We did not have a fallout; we just slowly drifted apart. I was like a piece of the mainland that through the ED's storms, broke off and became a lonely island. Thus, I spent many years alone, which fueled the ED and my social anxiety even more.

After that, it became much more difficult for me to interact with people. I was scared that I would sound dumb and that they would not like me. I wanted to make friends, but I was convinced that I would be unable to.

What has helped me is to remind myself of how much I want and need friendships. The times when I feel the happiest and are the most like myself are when I am spending time with other people. It is during these moments that I can get a sense of who I am outside of the ED. That is why the ED does not want you around others. It wants you all to itself so that the only thing you hear is its deceptive lies.

The ED does not want you to realize who you really are, because then you would recognize that you do not need it. You are a wonderful human being that is worthy and special and good enough exactly the way you are.

The fear of not being liked is not fact. Yes, there will always be people whom you do not see eye-to-eye with and those that you simply do not connect with, but you will see that there are individuals who will love you and cherish your friendship. However, in order to achieve this, you have to put yourself out there. I have begun reaching out to people I meet as well as trying to reconnect with friends from my past. Some of them do not work out, but a lot of them do. Having friends in your circle to show kindness to and receive kindness from is incredibly beneficial not just to ED recovery but also to feeling joy and purpose in life. Do not allow the ED to convince you that it is your only friend. It is not your friend, and there are so many wonderful true friends out in the world who are just waiting for you to reach out.

The ED tries to not only deceive you, but it causes you to deceive others, as well. Even though one of my biggest values is honesty, I have been led astray to lie to people about my behaviors. I either did not want to get in trouble, did not want others to think negatively of me, or I was just fearful about letting go of the ED. However, the only way to truly free yourself from this disorder is by being open and honest. Let your treatment team know what you are struggling with and what you need to work on. Let your supports know what they can look out for and what they can do to help. The more you keep things to yourself, the more the ED has control over you. In order to release this control, you have to let the truth out.

I have also found that sharing my recovery with others has helped encourage and inspire them to fight back to their own ED. I was being a model for others.

"Show yourself in all respects to be a model of good works, and in your teaching show integrity, dignity, and sound speech that cannot be condemned, so that an opponent [The ED] may be put to shame, having nothing evil to say about us" Titus 2:7-8.

For me, I receive great benefit from seeing people who have been through the tunnel that I am going through and have made it out to the other side. The road may still be bumpy for them sometimes, but they have the light. It shows me that victory is possible. Even when it feels like there is no way out, seeing someone who did succeed gives me the strength to keep trying.

"In the same way, let your light shine before others, so that they may see your good works and give glory to your Father who is in heaven" Matthew 5:16. My goal is to give back and be that light for others just as many have done for me. Many people have helped to encourage me and build me up, and I long to do the same for others. "Therefore encourage one another and build one another up, just as you are doing" 1 Thessalonians 5:11.

Not only does recovering from the ED allow us to help those who are struggling with an eating disorder, but it also allows us to help others by fulfilling our life's purpose. You DO have good things to give to the world, and do not let anything hold you back from doing that. "Do not withhold good from those to whom it is due, when it is in your power to do it" Proverbs 3:27.

We all have a purpose in life that is meant to better the world and those in it. If we do not take actions towards fulfilling our purpose, then all of the individuals whom we could have been able to help will be without. Our helpful actions will be seriously hindered if we allow the ED to stick around.

And, interactions with others lead to chain reactions. Even if we are only able to help one other person, that person can go on to help others. And, those people can help even more people, and so on. Thus, your good is being multiplied and shared with the world. A small spark can turn into a rampant blaze of good. But, just as starting a fire requires all the necessary equipment and tools, starting a spark of good requires us to be fueled with the necessary nutrition.

Sometimes it is challenging to create that spark, but we need to focus on the blaze and all the good that it can do. Even if you are not at the place yet where you can do recovery for yourself, do it for other people, and also for God. "And whatever you do, in word or deed, do everything in the name of the Lord Jesus, giving thanks to God the Father through him" Colossians 3:17. Focus on how your recovery can help others and how it is rooted in kindness. Focus on the difference you could make if you were not held back. Focus on what God thinks of you and what He desires for you and your life.

If you are not at the place yet to do it for yourself, that's completely okay. Focus on what motivators you do have and let the internal self-motivation grow over time. Trust me, it will. I have had many times where I was only doing this for other people. When you begin to realize the true benefits of recovery, you will start to want it for yourself. Recovery is a beautiful thing, and it is far greater than life in the ED.

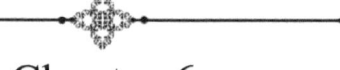

Chapter 6
Goodness

Goodness. We have been called by God to do good and be Christ-like in our actions. Even though our salvation comes from faith, we as Christ followers should still desire to spread good and share the love of Jesus with others.

However, no matter how much we love Jesus and try to live for Him, we will be hindered if we allow the ED to have any part of our lives. The ED's goal is not good, but destruction. Listening to it and its commands lead people towards paths that stray away from this good.

For me, the ED shifted my focus. I spent all my time and energy into worrying about myself and what I did not have or what I had that was not good enough. I was preoccupied by all the flaws and blemishes that I perceived my body to have, as well as what was wrong with my internal self and personality. It was as if my mind had a filter and all I could see was what was wrong with me.

This type of focus in no way benefitted me. It simply made me more anxious, depressed, and ashamed. I wanted to hide from the world, and I wanted to hide from myself. Instead of going out into the world and spreading good, all I wanted to do was curl up into a ball and shout hate towards myself.

I have found that rather than focusing on myself and what I do not have, it is far more beneficial for us to focus on others and what we can give. We are to seek God and righteousness in all that we do. "But seek first the kingdom of God and his righteousness, and all these things will be added to you" Matthew 6:33. This is the only way to fill the void and provide true fulfillment. Things of this world cannot give us what our souls desire. Our souls are at peace when we look to God and consider what we can do to serve Him and His children. "Set your minds on things that are above, not on things that are on earth" Colossians 3:2.

All of us have a purpose here on this earth. None of us are worthless; we all deserve to live and fulfill that purpose. However, in order to live life to the fullest, we cannot let the ED hold us back. "Do not be overcome by evil, but overcome evil with good" Romans 12:21. The ED is the evil darkness that is trying to control us. The only way to break this darkness is by lighting a light of good. We need to continue to do good and to do the next right thing. Instead of giving in, we must hold fast to our recovery mindset. "Let love be genuine. Abhor what is evil; hold fast to what is good" Romans 12:9.

Something that I did to help myself hang on to my recovery mindset was to write myself a letter. When my recovery mindset was the strongest and I had vigorous motivation, I wrote down all the reasons why I wanted to do this. Then, if my motivation ever began to wane, I would read the letter and remind myself of these things. Since the ED often tries to create a fog and hide our motivation, this is a way of turning on the flashlight and seeing past that.

In my letter, I included reminders as to how I felt in the ED. I was not happy. I was not at peace. I did not have the energy to do any of the things that I enjoyed or felt passionate about. I constantly felt poorly, and I was continually bombarded by threats and concerns brought about from my treatment providers and loved ones. I did not have any hobbies or friends, and I was hurting my family. I felt so alone. I felt trapped. All in all, I was miserable.

I also reminded myself of my goals. I wanted to be able to build those relationships back and acquire new ones. I wanted to be able to have fun and enjoy life's beautiful moments. I wanted to be able to eat a meal like a "normal person" and not be consumed by the fear, guilt, and anxiety that the ED wanted me to feel. I wanted to go to college and have my dream career. I wanted to help others and fulfill my purpose. I wanted a life!

None of these goals are possible while remaining trapped in the ED. The only way to achieve them is by breaking free by holding fast to good and avoiding what is wrong. I had to overcome the evil ED with good.

I have also found that the ED tried to shift my love to hate. I spent so much time focusing on how I hated my body and how I hated myself. I was convinced that every part of me was wrong or flawed in some way, and that it made me a worthless creature. But, my appearance does not define who I am. What matters is inward goodness. Rather than focusing on self-hatred and the loathing of food, we are to focus on love and goodness. "Finally, brothers, whatever is true, whatever is honorable, whatever is just, whatever is pure, whatever is lovely, whatever is commendable, if there is any excellence, if there is anything worthy of praise, think about these things" Philippians 4:8.

Instead of focusing on what is wrong with myself, I have found that I benefit much more from focusing on what I can do right. Instead of using my time in a way that is harmful, I devote that time and energy into benefiting those for whom Christ died, because that is what God wants us to do. "Commit your work to the Lord, and your plans will be established" Proverbs 16:3. And, I cannot help others when I am killing myself.

Being in treatment caused me to be around a lot of people who were struggling. At first, I would keep to myself and wallow in my own depression. I sat out of group activities and games, and I kept quiet during mealtime conversations. Instead of choosing joy and love, I chose to remain in my anger and fear. But, that neither helped me nor anyone else. It just increased my suffering and did nothing to help others who were trapped, themselves.

I found that as I came out of my shell and let go of the rope of depression, I not only helped myself, but I was able to help those with whom I interacted with. I was able to form meaningful connections, and I could share goodness with others.

Since it takes me a while to warm up to people who I do not know well and am not close with, I used a method that was most comfortable for me. I would write down little encouraging notes and hand them to my peers who needed them most. Sometimes I would give it to them directly, and other times I would just place it somewhere for them to find later. These small gestures may seem insignificant, but they actually had a major impact. My peers were able to benefit from words of encouragement or inspiration. And, even if the words that I wrote were not especially helpful, it always seemed to brighten their day to know that someone cared.

This act helped me to not only make it through the day, but to look forward to the days to come. The more I wrote encouraging notes, the more I started to believe that what I was writing was applicable to myself. Since I believe in hope for every single person on this earth, maybe I can extend that towards myself. And, the more I helped others, my desire to live and recover increased, because I felt like I had a purpose. I had something I could do that would be beneficial and meaningful, and for that I wanted to stick around.

I encourage you to find a goal that is for good and contributes to what you are passionate about. Pursue it! Go at it and give it your all! "Whatever your hand finds to do, do it with your might" Ecclesiastes 9:10. This is what helps me feel like my life is meaningful. This is what motivates me to get out of bed every morning and tackle the challenges that come my way. This is what reminds me of who I am and what I care about. I am not my disorder, and neither are you.

When I began to give up the ED and become myself again, I realized that I had to rediscover who I was. For so long, I had been my disorder, and it became my identity. It had become the subject of all my thoughts, and it had been the guide for all of my actions. My interests were its interests, and my hobbies were its behaviors. The thought of who I was outside of the ED left me with a major question mark.

You may have noticed that I consistently refer to the ED as "the" instead of "my". That is because this is my way of separating myself from it. Yes, it does often lead me towards its behaviors, but it is not who I am. I am Noël. The ED was something that I struggled with and still sometimes do, but it is not a part of my identity. I am so much more, and you are, too.

Discovering your true joys and passions is so essential to learning who you are. It helps you come up with what will make life worth living for you. This meaningful life is what helps us persist even when storm after storm blow our way. It is what helps us keep going despite our weaknesses and desires to surrender. It shows us that there are things in life that provide us with fulfillment that are far better than the temporary high received from engaging in an ED behavior.

When I began to give up my old ways of thinking and acting, I had to find out what I really liked. Many of my old hobbies prior to the ED no longer resonated with me, because I had become a different person. Some of my interests were similar, but a lot had changed. I had grown up, and I was in a new phase of my life.

So, since I had PLENTY of down time in treatment, this gave me the opportunity to discover new passions. I had a wide variety of art, games, and literature at my disposal, as well as stories and experiences from many different people, so I decided to try things out. I pursued topics that piqued my interest, as well as trying activities that I never would have considered had I not been in that setting. Each time I found something that made me feel like a person and separate from the ED, that is how I knew that this was a passion of mine. If it brought me even a small moment where I felt freedom from the ED, I knew that was something for me.

I am honestly still in the process of discovering who I am, and that's okay. The discovery process is a part of living, and it's fun! Life is so much bigger than the box that the ED tries to squeeze us into. Take chances, have fun, and enjoy the ride!

One hobby of mine that I developed is writing. I love using my creativity and ideas to write in a way that is meaningful to others. However, the judgmental and critical side of myself was convinced that it would not let me win. I believe this is the ED's way of making us feel less than and drawing us back to it. If we get caught in the lies that we are not good enough, the ED has a greater chance of convincing us that it has the solution. "You're not good enough, but if you lost this much weight and ate this certain way…"

I was bombarded by fears that I was inferior. It criticized everything I did and who I was as a person. "Your writings are stupid." "No one would ever want to read what you wrote." "You're a failure and should just give up!"

I did give up for a while. In fact, after I began this very book, I put it aside because the ED led me to believe that it would never amount to anything. And, giving up on my ED recovery book even led me to believe that recovery itself could never be possible.

However, with the help of my therapist, I realized that my book does not need to be perfect. No one, except God, is capable of perfection, so I cannot hold these unrealistic standards for myself. I cannot let my fears keep me from doing good and achieving my goal of helping others. Writing is something that I am passionate about and brings me joy, and sharing it with others could possibly bring them joy. I did not want to let evil overcome this good, so I persisted. That is why you are able to read this book today.

Whenever you start wanting to give up on recovery, or anything else good in your life, remind yourself of your goals and passions and what you are fighting for. What makes you smile? What gives you a sense of meaning and purpose? What allows you to truly feel like yourself? No matter what the naysayers inside or outside of your head say, listen to the small voice telling you that this is what you are meant to do. God will be with you, and He will guide you through the struggles and help you make decisions for good. I encourage you to make a daily commitment to live your life for good. You will be surprised as to how much this will benefit your recovery and your life.

Chapter 7
Faithfulness

Faithfulness. I am very blessed to have had the gift of growing up in a strong Christian home. Ever since I can remember, I have been praying to God and singing His songs of praise and worship. I knew that Jesus loved me, and that God is my amazing Father and Lord. Throughout my time growing up when I learned about faithfulness, I never imagined that I would have an issue with it. Of course I would serve the Lord; who else would I worship? I would never bow down to a wooden idol!

However, I have learned that the ED is a form of idol. It is something that strays us away from God and all His truths. It demands our complete devotion and leaves little to no room for anything else.

When I was in my worst in my battle against the ED, God was slipping out of the picture. I would pray to Him, but my motive was in the wrong place. Instead of praying with the Lord's will in mind, I would ask for weight-loss or some other ED goal. Instead of studying the Bible, I would study nutrition facts and tricks to lose weight fast. And when I did read in the Bible, the ED always found a way to twist God's Word and make me think that it was reinforcing the ED. Instead of hearing God's truth, I found ways to fit the verses into what I wanted them to mean so that they encouraged ED rules and behaviors. I still was a believer, but I was slowly drifting away.

"Put to death therefore what is earthly in you: sexual immorality, impurity, passion, evil desire, and covetousness, which is idolatry" Colossians 3:5. The Bible tells us to put away sinful and unhealthy behaviors. Giving in to the ED meant that I was focusing on unhealthy behaviors and longing for things that were not beneficial to me and were in fact hurting me. The ED was causing me to do wrong and act in ways that were not Christ-like. I was letting the ED be my idol.

This is a concept that was personally very difficult for me to accept. Like I said, for a long time, I was perfectly convinced that I was doing all the right things. The ED had deceived me into believing that it was right and anything contrary to it was wrong and immoral. However, when I began to realize all the destructiveness that it was causing towards me and those around me, I recognized that the ED is not a good thing. And, when I realized how much devotion I was giving to it versus other aspects of my life, I saw that this was a major problem.

One activity I did in treatment was create a pie chart on how my time was divided up. We were told to incorporate various day to day tasks as well as activities that the ED causes us to engage in, whether that is actual behaviors, or things such as rumination, worrying, and planning. When attempting to do the activity, my perfectionism wasted a lot of time trying to ensure I divided my time on the pie chart completely accurately. But, when I was finally able to push this fear aside, I was able to actually do the activity. I honestly reflected on what my life had become: not on what I wanted it to be or what I thought the "correct" answer was. I saw how small my time with God had gotten and how large sections related to the ED was. The ED had become the major focus of my life. Even when I was not acting on a behavior, it was still in the front of my mind and was consuming and controlling everything. That was a wakeup call.

As Christians, we know that our devotion should be to the Lord God Almighty, not to the ED. The Lord has done much for us and deserves/desires/demands our complete devotion. "You shall love the Lord your God with all your heart and with all your soul and with all your might" Deuteronomy 6:5. He should be our number one. "You shall have no other gods before me" Exodus 20:3.

The ED tries to squeeze its way into our heart and soul, and once it is there, its goal is to take over and become number one. It wants to dominate our lives and become, essentially, our god.

Do not let the ED be your god! Not only does it stray us away from God, but it leads us towards harm. It tries to sound wise and helpful, but its commands are actually the opposite. There are three verses I have found that describe the ED's faulty commands:

> "So do not be attracted by strange, new ideas. Your strength comes from God's grace, not from rules about food, which don't help those who follow them" Hebrews 13:9 (NLT)

> "If with Christ you died to the elemental spirits of the world, why, as if you were still alive in the world, do you submit to regulations - 'Do not handle, Do not taste, Do not touch' (referring to things that all perish as they are used) - according to human precepts and

teachings? These have indeed an appearance of wisdom in promoting self-made religion and asceticism and severity to the body, but they are of no value in stopping the indulgence of the flesh" Colossians 2:20-23

"They will say it is wrong to be married and wrong to eat certain foods. But God created those foods to be eaten with thanks by faithful people who know the truth. Since everything God created is good, we should not reject any of it but receive it with thanks. For we know it is made acceptable by the word of God and prayer" 1 Timothy 4:3-5 (NLT)

As these verses describe, the ED tries to come up with rules and regulations that are the complete opposite of truth. Rather than accepting food with thanksgiving and joy, which is what we are meant to do, it tries to tell us to not eat or that we must follow certain food rules. These rules focus on depriving ourselves or treating ourselves harshly. They sound wise and helpful, and since the ED is very convincing, we believe it. However, we receive no benefit from these commands. They do not give us what we need.

The only One who can provide us with what we truly need is Jesus Christ. "Jesus said to her, 'Everyone who drinks of this water will be thirsty again, but whoever drinks of the water that I will give him will never be thirsty again. The water that I will give him will become in him a spring of water welling up to eternal life'" John 4:13-14.

Even though I thought that the way I was treating food and my body would give me satisfaction, it never did. I never felt like I was eating the correct way. I never thought that my body looked good enough. And, I never thought that I was good enough. Instead of feeling proud of what I had accomplished, I was driven by a need for more, more, more! I constantly felt a void inside, and the ED failed to fill it.

Only Jesus can give us the love, joy, peace, security, strength, comfort, and everything else that our souls desire. The way to fill the void that you are seeking to fill is by seeking God and being faithful to Him. "A faithful man will abound with blessings" Proverbs 28:20. As you continue to let God more into your heart, He will fill it with all the fruits of the spirit. Instead of being emotionally empty, you will finally be able to feel satisfied.

So, how does one grow closer to God? The two biggest actions that help me are prayer and exploring God's Word. It can be especially helpful to link the two. Before I sit down to read the Bible, I pray that God will speak to me and tell me what He wants me to hear. I then read with open eyes and an open heart. Whatever God tells me, I must be willing to accept and willing to do. "This Book of the Law shall not depart from your mouth, but you shall meditate on it day and night, so that you may be careful to do according to all that is written in it. For then you will make your way prosperous, and then you will have good success" Joshua 1:8.

What I mean by an open heart is that you must be willing to accept what God says to you; you cannot brush it aside or dismiss it. Wherever He guides us to or away from, we must be willing to obey. This also means that we cannot distort the words to fit into what we want them to mean, like I used to do. Rather than shaping His Word around our (or the ED's) beliefs, we need to conform our beliefs around His Word.

An open heart also means that your heart is open to God and closed to everything else. The ED will work hard to squeeze its way in there. For me, it always tried to have me hold on to seemingly insignificant behaviors. As long as I was meeting my nutritional needs, why would it matter how I did that? I would hang on to various food rules and rituals because I thought they were fine.

However, this was the ED's way of getting into my heart. Then, the snowball effect occurred. One small behavior led to another small behavior and another small behavior, and then eventually a bigger behavior and then an even bigger behavior. I no longer was engaging in insignificant behaviors; I had entered a full-blown relapse.

The truth is that any bit of the ED we hold on to can be extremely detrimental to our health. It may not seem significant at first but trust me when I say that it matters. Denying this truth will only lead to your downfall.

The only way to successfully conquer the ED is by knowing the truth. This was a struggle for me. I constantly had medical professionals and therapists try to ingrain into my brain the facts about the ED and why I should not believe it. They tried to explain how its rules are faulty and harmful as well as how the ED was negatively affecting my body. However, because the ED had such a tight grip on me, I did not believe them. I was convinced that I was the exception to this science. Maybe that was true for everyone else, but not for me.

Thankfully, we do not need to focus on science. Instead, we can listen to God. In His Word, we find His numerous promises that we can put our faith in. We can find what truly matters in life. And, we can find God's view of us and how He loves us for who we are.

God loves us; the ED does not. God satisfies; the ED increases our longing. God gives us peace; the ED adds to our worries. God heals; the ED destroys. God will lead us to a beautiful future, while the ED leads only to death.

Sometimes when I was in the ED, I thought that I wanted death. Since I was having a miserable life, I just wanted to die. But, that is because I was not truly living. With the ED, I was barely existing. Trust me that outside of the ED there is a wonderful life, and it is worth living for. You can experience joy and fulfillment. I used to think it was not possible, but I have found that it is. There is only one way to get there, and that is by pursuing recovery.

God has placed each of us on this earth for a reason, and He has a specific time for when each of us are to go home. We may not understand why, but He does. Throughout the uncertainty and through the times of trial and tribulation, we can lean on God and trust Him to be with us. Even though we may wander astray, He will never leave us. He is forever faithful.

Recovery is not perfect and there will be difficult times. There will be times that we want to give up and times when we believe that we cannot possibly go on for another minute. The key is to stay faithful to the process. Commit to staying on the right path no matter what it takes. And when you are unsure as to what to do, because the ED will make things very difficult sometimes, seek truth. Whenever I come to a difficult recovery decision, I ask myself, "Is this what God wants for me or what the ED wants?" I encourage you to ask yourself this question as well, and choose the path that leads to abundant life. That abundant life is out there, and it is waiting for you.

Chapter 8
Gentleness

Gentleness. This chapter is devoted to being gentle to ourselves. Rather than tearing down our bodies in the way that the ED tries to have us do, we are to build up and strengthen our bodies, because they are temples of God. "Or do you not know that your body is a temple of the Holy Spirit within you, whom you have from God? You are not your own, for you were bought with a price. So glorify God in your body" 1 Corinthians 6:19-20.

When I was deep in the ED, I was blinded by what I was doing. I was fully convinced that altering my body was my way of repairing the temple. I thought that my striving to lose weight was doing the right thing by making myself better. However, changing my body only benefitted the ED. It did not help the Lord or advance my life's purpose. In fact, it took me further away from being able to fulfill that purpose.

Instead of giving me the strength to make a positive change, it caused me to barely have the strength to walk across the floor. Instead of letting me go out into the world to spread good, it caused me to go in and out of ERs and treatment centers. Instead of building up my confidence, it led me to feel even more insecure and to isolate. Instead of moving me closer to where I was meant to go, the ED actually led me in the opposite direction.

I was not focusing on what God wanted me to do with my body. Instead, I was completely ignoring Him by obeying the ED. I allowed the ED to tear up my body. And, if I had continued to follow it, it would have killed me.

But, my body is not my own; it is the Lord's. While I am watching over this body, I need to take care of it in the way that God wants me to, and I need to use it for Him. "I appeal to you therefore, brothers, by the mercies of God, to present your bodies as a living sacrifice, holy and acceptable to God, which is your spiritual worship" Romans 12:1.

The ED expects us to sacrifice our bodies to it. It wants us to give up everything that is important to us. No matter how much pain and suffering we experience, the ED demands that we, like slaves, continue to labor for it. If we fail to measure up to its standards, it punishes us with brutal beatings.

However, sacrificing ourselves to God is different. He is not a Master of hatred and cruelty, but of love. His desire for us to obey His commands is because He cares about and wants the best for us. He wants to keep us from evil and bring us towards good. And His command to sacrifice does not involve giving up meaningful things, but worldly things. God desires for us to set ourselves apart as holy and live for Him. And that includes keeping our bodily temples holy.

So, what does the phrase "my body is a temple" really mean? It means that we are valued vessels, and that Christ lives inside of us. "I have been crucified with Christ. It is no longer I who live, but Christ who lives in me. And the life I now live in the flesh I live by faith in the Son of God, who loved me and gave himself for me" Galatians 2:20.

We are important. We are important to Christ, and we are important to the purpose that we have the opportunity to fulfill while dwelling in this body. We are not run-down shacks that can be cleared away because we serve no purpose. Rather, we are beautiful temples that are treasured by God and have beautiful and special purposes.

And, just as the Lord is holy, and since He dwells in us, we must act in ways that are in accordance with Him. "Since we have these promises, beloved, let us cleanse ourselves from every defilement of body and spirit, bringing holiness to completion in the fear of God" 2 Corinthians 7:1. This is telling us that we need to cleanse ourselves from things that are harmful to us, and that includes the ED. We need to stop engaging in behaviors that are destructive to our bodies and stop listening to the lies that it tries to make us believe. Instead, we are to act in ways that are in accordance with who we are. We are not our disorders. We are beloved children of God, and we deserve to be treated with love and respect.

Rather than hating our bodies, we can show ourselves the love and respect that we deserve. "No one hates his own body but feeds and cares for it, just as Christ cares for the church" Ephesians 5:29 (NLT). God cares about us, and He wants us to be gentle to ourselves and show ourselves this same love and care.

The most basic way to do this is by meeting our needs, and one universal need is food. Every single living being is in need of food in order to survive. Food helps us to live, function, flourish, and blossom. Depriving yourself of this or engaging with it in an unhealthy way is not taking care of yourself. Instead of building yourself up, it is a way of tearing yourself down.

God wants us to eat in a way that properly nourishes our bodies so that we have the strength and energy to live our lives. And, all human beings need food, regardless of their body types. This means that no matter where you are on the BMI scale or any other weight chart, you still need sufficient nutrition.

No matter what you or others say about your body, you still need food. No matter what size clothing you wear, you still need food. No matter what the scale or the tape measurer says, you still need food. And not just enough to live by, but the amount that your beautiful, amazing, fantastic body needs!

I used to be convinced that my body was too big and that I did not deserve to receive nutrients above the absolute bare minimum. So, I deprived myself. I lost the weight, but I also lost my health and every bit of contentment in life. I lost the things that were important to me and the people who were important to me. Instead of gaining benefits, I lost nearly everything that I once had. Instead of improving my quality of life, I destroyed it.

This was difficult for me to acknowledge, but after all the loss that the ED had caused, I could no longer deny it. This does not mean that I do not still struggle with my body. I still am not satisfied with my body size, but my appearance no longer determines my actions. I have more important things in my life to devote my attention towards. I am working on accepting my body and focusing on what it can do rather than what it looks like.

And, in order for my body to do good, I have to give it the proper fuel.

One way that I have found to help myself with accepting my body is by looking at it from a different perspective. How do I view others in different body shapes? I do not look down upon others due to their weight, nor do I feel as if they need to be deprived. Every human being is a worthy child of God, and every human being both needs and deserves food.

For example, I am a proud cat mom of five lovely kitties. Just as humans have different bodies, so do cats, and my cats all have different shapes and sizes. Some are in smaller bodies, and the others are much larger. Still, that does not stop me from meeting their nutritional needs. They all deserve to receive care and adequate nutrition. We can apply this same concept to ourselves. Just as I love each of my cats, God loves each and every one of us. And, He does not want us to be neglecting ourselves of this care.

Looking a different way does not make us any less worthy or deserving. God would love you the same if you were double your current weight or half of it. The important thing is whether you are nourishing your body so that it can be and do all that it is meant to. Are your eating habits helping you live life for yourself and for God, or is it stopping you? That's what is important. Whatever weight in which you experience life abundantly is the right weight for you.

Another way that we can be gentle to ourselves is by engaging in enjoyable activities. This may not sound important, but it is actually a valuable form of self-care. I have found that when I fully immerse myself into a conversation or a fun hobby, that is when I truly discover who I am apart from the ED. It helps to push aside the gloom and doom, and it causes me to feel like I am really living. Instead of being negative or apathetic towards life, it enables me to have a more positive and joyful outlook.

I am not going to lie; this is hard. I know that when I am depressed, all I want to do is shut down and be by myself. (Although, I am not truly by myself. Instead, I am being drawn closer and closer to the ED.) I have found, though, that when I do take that chance and go all in, I never regret it. In order to swim, we first must get into the water. That's taking the chance. Then we must paddle and stroke and give it our all. When we do not fully try, that is when we sink.

I also sometimes struggle with giving myself time to relax because I feel guilty for not being productive. But, everyone needs a break. Even God took a day of rest. Genesis 2:2 tells us, "And on the seventh day God finished his work that he had done, and he rested on the seventh day from all his work that he had done." Surely if He can, we can, too.

Pushing yourself too hard does not benefit you any. Rather than resulting in increased productivity, it actually begins to wear you out. As a high achiever, I once was all work and no play. How could I relax when so much needed to be done? And, even if things did not have to be done, I still felt as if they were more important than lying around doing nothing! Unfortunately, this led to me be tired and irritable, my performance started struggling, and I just was not happy.

I have found that giving myself a break gives my body and mind an opportunity to recharge. It gives me that little boost and pick-me-up to get back on track and keep going. It also brings more joy into my life, which positively affects so many aspects of what I am able to do and how I am able to function. Instead of doing what I feared, it did the opposite.

The same is true with punishment. I was convinced that me punishing myself would motivate me to be better. Some examples of punishment from my own life include restriction, obsessive exercise, purging, self-harm, and negative self-talk, but it can also include any other destructive habit that the ED tries to convince you to do. I thought that I was helping better myself, but I was only hurting myself even more.

For me, the restriction was meant as a punishment for looking a certain way. I believed that I was a horrible person for allowing my body to get so large, and I needed to do something to change it. However, God created my body and chose for it to be this way. We all have different set points assigned by God. What this means is that God designed a specific range for each of us which is where our bodies naturally sit when we meet our nutritional needs. Even if we eat a little extra some days or are ill and unable to eat enough on others, our bodies will still stay roughly around that spot.

When I first heard of set points, it made no sense to me. I was convinced that my treatment team came up with a number and was going to force me to get there because that is what they thought was best for me. However, after much petition on my end, they explained the process as to how they figured out where my restored body would be, and I was able to have faith in the process. I may not like where my body rests, but that is what God created for me. I should not punish myself for being the way that God wants me to be. Instead, I can learn to embrace it, or at least accept it.

The obsessive exercise and purging were used as punishments for what I had eaten. I felt guilt or disgust over what I had put inside of my body. But, every body needs food, and I am not an exception. We can also have peace in knowing that the Designer designed our bodies to know exactly what to do with what we eat. Our bodies know how to break food down and use it in the way that we need. We should not punish ourselves for giving our bodies vital nutrients. Instead, we can say "thank you".

It may sound bizarre to thank our bodies for eating, and you most likely will not feel very thankful at first. However, the more you continue to repeat this practice, you may begin to notice that a tiny part of you is grateful. It may be most helpful to start small. You can consider those who grew the foods or prepared the meal. You can be thankful for the opportunity to spend with loved ones while eating the food. You can focus on what the food allows your body to do. And, maybe you even enjoy (or have a slight likeness of) the taste. Allow your gratitude to slowly grow over time until you can thank YOURSELF for eating.

Another form of punishment for me was self-harm. I used self-harm as a means of punishing myself whenever I did something "bad" or "not good enough". However, no human being is perfect. As long as we give it our best, that is all that we could possibly do. Rather than punishing ourselves, we can feel proud that we gave it our all, because that is a win.

An activity that I found to be helpful is writing down things I do well each day. Like the gratitude list mentioned earlier in this book, I increasingly added on the amount that I would write each day. And, you do not have to fully believe it. Let that grow over time. Just make sure you acknowledge what you do well, or at least what you do "not so horribly". These do not have to be major achievements. It could be something as simple as putting in effort towards a task or getting out of bed in the morning. The reality is that these "simple" achievements are actually efforts worth being proud of. Every effort deserves to be acknowledged and celebrated.

It took a lot of time and practice, but this truly helped me identify that I am not a complete failure. I am able to accomplish good and I do live in a way that is worth being proud of. I do not deserve to beat up on myself, and neither do you.

This beating up on myself, or negative self-talk, was meant to encourage me to do better in the future. But, it did not build me up; it tore me down and nearly destroyed me. Instead of improving and feeling like a better person, I ended up feeling even worse about myself. I tried countless therapy techniques to try to counter these core beliefs, but nothing was believable. I was encouraged to tell myself what I would tell a friend, but I was not my own friend. How could I speak to myself like a friend when I was my own worst enemy?

I then was introduced to an activity where I was encouraged to imagine what a compassionate friend would say to me during distressing situations. At first, I was stumped. At that point in my life, I did not really have any friends. Since I was expected to come up with something, I continued to think, and then it hit me: Who is a more compassionate friend than Jesus?! He loves me through it all, and no matter how many times I struggle or fall short, He comforts and encourages me. What a friend we have in Jesus! Now, when I notice that I am speaking cruelly to myself, I pause and ask, "What would Jesus say to me in this situation?"

If you cannot come up with something, just look in God's Word and review the countless encouragements that He gives. Just as Jesus encouraged His disciples and other people that He interacted with during His time on this earth, so does He encourage us today. And know that God is love. Everything He says and does stems from this beautiful, unconditional love.

I just want to emphasize that this is my own experience. Maybe the "What Would You Say to a Friend?" Activity works for you, and that is great; go for it. Recovery is about doing what works for you. However, if you are in the same place as I was, then this is a good method to try. I pray that as you continue to practice gentleness towards yourself in both actions and words, you will slowly begin to build your relationship with yourself and that you will become your own friend. It takes time, but you will get there. And be gentle with yourself throughout the process. It is just that- a process- and as long as you try your best, that is enough.

You are enough, and you deserve gentleness. Take care of yourself, because you are a wonderful, precious, worthy child of God.

Chapter 9
Self-Control

Self-control. One reason why people cling to their ED is because it gives them a sense of control. The world is filled with a lot of chaos and situations that we have no influence over. Negative events can overwhelm us and cause us to feel like we need something. So, we resort to the ED where we try to obtain that sense of control. "There is a way that seems right to a man, but its end is the way to death" Proverbs 16:25. The ED helps us feel good temporarily and as if we have achieved that control. However, this is only a feeling. We are not the ones in control; the ED is.

When I first developed the ED, I thought that I was so amazing for being able to control what I ate. I felt like I was a strong individual with willpower. I was able to avoid giving in to temptations and I was changing myself for the better, or so I thought. However, as I began to plunge deeper and deeper into the ED, that feeling went away. Even times when I wanted to do more, I couldn't. I even scheduled "cheat days", but I was too weak to actually have them when the time came around. And, when the threat of going to a treatment center came up, I was unable to stop my behaviors and do what needed to be done to avoid it. I went from being confident in my control to completely spiraling out of control.

In following the ED, rather than gaining control, we ultimately give all the control that we once had over to it. It hops in the driver seat of our life, and we are pushed aside to the back. It controls the turns and stops, while we merely hang on for the ride. We have nothing, and the ED has everything.

Unfortunately, the ED is not the one that we should allow this control to be transferred to. As I have continually emphasized, it cannot help us. It does not give us what we need or desire. The only One that can do this is God. Instead of giving control to the ED, we should turn it over to God. Let Him be the Rule-maker through whom your actions are in accordance with. "Do not be conformed to this world, but be transformed by the renewal of your mind, that by testing you may discern what is the will of God, what is good and acceptable and perfect" Romans 12:2.

The worldly ED wants us to conform to its ways and have control over us, but we cannot let evil win. "Do not swerve to the right or to the left; turn your foot away from evil" Proverbs 4:27. We must continue straight along the path of recovery and put away the ED, because the path of recovery is the only road that leads to life. "For if you live according to the flesh you will die, but if by the Spirit you put to death the deeds of the body, you will live" Romans 8:13.

The ED tried to tell me that it would give me a life worth living. If I followed certain rules and got my body to look a certain way, I would be happy, it claimed. However, I never was. I may have liked my body more, but I never liked it. Plus, my preoccupation with how my body looked and with food only increased. And, in all other areas of my life, I was more anxious, depressed, and miserable. I literally felt as if I had nothing except the ED, and all the ED did was abuse me, both physically and mentally.

The ED used to convince me that I was not happy yet, but I would get there. If I just engaged in more behaviors and lost more weight, then I would be happy. It took a lot of time to accept this, but I now recognize that there is never enough. Doing more behaviors does not lead to more happiness; it leads to death. I came close to that many times. I did not realize it then, but that was because my critical thinking skills were so clouded by all the lies of the ED. You may not believe it, but I promise you that the threat is REAL!

The ED's ultimate goal is not for us to be thin and beautiful or to eat the perfect amount of food in the perfect way. Trying to achieve this nonexistent perfection is its means of bringing us where it wants us: death. With the ED in the driver's seat, our destination is not paradise, but a deadly car accident.

The ED lies. I often call it the Evil Deceiver, because that is exactly what it is. It deceives us about every part of life, and its intentions are wicked and cruel. So, we must constantly be on the lookout for this. "I appeal to you, brothers, to watch out for those who cause divisions and create obstacles contrary to the doctrine that you have been taught; avoid them. For such persons do not serve our Lord Christ, but their own appetites, and by smooth talk and flattery they deceive the hearts of the naïve" Romans 16:17-18.

The ED lies about so many things. Through its many lies, it tries to change our beliefs about food. I went from loving food to absolutely hating it all because of how the ED twisted my brain. Instead of looking forward to food-centered occasions and celebrations, they became sources of extreme panic and distress. Instead of savoring the taste and experience of eating, I was consumed by the fears in my head. My favorite foods became my biggest fear foods, and hardly anything was safe.

But, I now know that this is not reality. All foods are good and are blessings for us to enjoy. How I see my body is not reality, either. Body dysmorphia is REAL! It distorts how we perceive our body, causing us to see ourselves through a lens that no one else sees. I personally still do not understand it, and oftentimes I try to fight it. However, I have to put my faith in trusted others that care about me to let me know the truth of the matter. I also must remind myself that how I look does not matter. Even if I do look the way that my brain tells me I look, that is okay, too. The ED will try to say that weight is important, but that is yet another deception. My weight is not an important factor in who I am. It is just one tiny component that makes up my body, and it in no way affects my worth or who I am as a person.

The ED lies about what is important, and it lies about who we are. What is important is not how we see ourselves, but how God sees us. And who we are is children of God. We are not owned by the ED; we belong to God.

You can regain control over your life. Even when the ED tempts us and tries to make us act in a certain way, we can stand strong. God promises that we will never be tempted beyond what we can handle. "No temptation has overtaken you that is not common to man. God is faithful, and he will not let you be tempted beyond your ability, but with the temptation he will also provide the way of escape, that you may be able to endure it" 1 Corinthians 10:13.

The ED's temptations are often very strong, and this may cause us to feel as if we do not stand a chance, but we do. The Lord has equipped each and every one of us with all that we need to fight our battles. "Therefore take up the whole armor of God, that you may be able to withstand in the evil day, and having done all, to stand firm. Stand therefore, having fastened on the belt of truth, and having put on the breastplate of righteousness, and, as shoes for your feet, having put on the readiness given by the gospel of peace. In all circumstances take up the shield of faith, with which you can extinguish all the flaming darts of the evil one; and take the helmet of salvation, and the sword of the Spirit, which is the word of God" Ephesians 6:13-17. With the truth, righteousness, readiness, peace, faith, and God's promises, we can combat the ED and win our battle for good!

The truth reveals the deceptions of the ED. Righteousness will keep us away from the ED's path and on the one that leads to abundant life. Readiness will prepare us for whatever the ED throws our way. Peace will help us stand firm through the storm, and it will give us the comfort that we need to overcome our anxieties and fears. Keeping our faith grounded in God will leave little room for the ED to creep in. God's many promises give us hope and assurance that everything will be okay, and that God will be with us through it all. With this armor, we are ready.

Also in treatment, we learn different skills and techniques to help us fight these battles, so I will include some of the ones that I personally find most beneficial.

Again, these are the ones that work for me. You may have completely different strategies that work for you. If you do, go for it. These are just a few techniques for you to try to see what sticks.

I also encourage you to come up with a few of your top go-to skills and techniques that help you when you are in the midst of the ED's strongest temptations. Write them down on a card or on the memo app on your phone. Just put it somewhere that you will have easy access to and will see frequently. Then when you notice yourself starting to struggle, turn to the list. You cannot just write the list and then abandon it; you must actively use it. It takes work to win your battles, so make sure to put in the work. It is worth it, I promise.

One of my favorites skills that I learned from treatment centers is assessing the pros and cons of a decision. Acknowledge what the benefits are as well as what the downsides are to whatever decision you are contemplating. It is important to write these down in a chart so that you can visually see and assess which is the best route to take. When deciding, make sure not to merely pay attention to the length of each list, but you must recognize the importance of each point. For example, in treatment, I have often made pros and cons lists for whether or not I should engage in an ED behavior, and normally I am able to make the pros list pretty lengthy. But, if I connect with my values, I realize that the cons are more significant to me. Acting on a behavior may help temporarily in the short term, but it brings an immense amount of pain in the long term, and it goes against many of the things that are truly important to me. Remember, do not let the ED control your decisions; let your values and God's Word be your guide.

Another technique that sometimes works for me is fact checking. I say "sometimes" because when I am listening to the ED, it is very hard to see the truth. When the ED is roaring strong, no logic sounds factual to me. Still, I have found that if I repeatedly tell myself a certain fact and why it is true, it will start to seep in. This, for me, takes a really long time. The important thing is to not give up. Sometimes I have been convinced that I would never believe certain concepts, but I am slowly starting to. Time and effort really do play an important role in overcoming whatever trial we may face.

Also, regarding fact checking, it is helpful to have a trusted support person assist you in reminding you of the truth. When all I can see is the ED, it is hard for me to come up with a logical counter response. But, having an outside person help with this can be incredibly beneficial. They can provide you with the truth, as well as asking you questions to get you to recognize the truth. "Tell me why you feel this way?" "Is this you, or the ED?" "What does God say about this?" Have a conversation with your support people and tell them what works specifically for you. This may change over time, and that's okay. Just be sure to continue to talk with these people about what they can do to best support you.

Support people are wonderful ways to help individuals stay on track with recovery. Try to accumulate as many of these trusted, supportive people as you can. This can include treatment team members, family, friends, church community members, and anyone else who loves you and desires for you to pursue a recovery focused life. And do not shut them out! The times when you feel most inclined to isolate from them are the moments in which you need them the most.

Again, I want to emphasize that using skills and combating the ED is often really difficult to do. You do not need to feel discouraged when the battle knocks you down. That's okay. Everyone falls sometimes. The important thing is that you get back up and try again. As long as you keep doing this, you will learn to walk the path of recovery. Then, you will be able to run. God will give you the strength to overcome this disorder. "For the grace of God has appeared, bringing salvation for all people, training us to renounce ungodliness and worldly passions, and to live self-controlled, upright, and godly lives in the present age" Titus 2:11-12.

You CAN renounce ungodliness and say "no" to the ED, and you CAN reclaim your life. Just don't lose hope and don't give up. Keep fighting the good fight. One day God will help you win this war. The ED does not have to control you any longer!

Conclusion

I hope that in this book, you have found meaningful verses and insight that benefit you in your or a loved one's recovery. These are just things that I have learned throughout my journey. To be honest, my journey is far from over. I still have a lot to learn and many more skills that I need to develop, but I am relying on God and trusting Him to provide me with these when the time is right.

I can honestly say that I feel more like myself now than I have in a very long time, and I continue to discover more of myself each and every day. I wake up each morning ready to experience the beautiful life that God has so lovingly blessed me with the opportunity of experiencing. This is not saying that I do not ever struggle. I still have difficult moments, some harder than others, but I work through them. I make daily commitments to fight this battle, and I am moving closer and closer to the point of full self-acceptance.

In the meantime, I continue to meet my needs. I meet with my treatment team and have an open and honest relationship with them. I have a meal plan that is designed to make sure I receive the foods I need, and I am actively growing closer to God to absorb all His spiritual fruits. This nourishment is what strengthens me and prepares me for what life throws my way. I encourage you to also nourish your body and soul, because this is the only way to achieve recovery and freedom.

Recovery does not look the same for everyone, and there is no magic guide to walk you through the process. Each person requires a unique treatment approach that is best suited for their individual needs. However, in order to achieve true healing, we all need God. God is the Ultimate Healer who loves you and wants you to reach out to Him. Seek Him and allow Him to guide you through this process.

Recovery IS possible and it IS worth it. It will be a difficult journey, but if you seek Him, God will use the fruits of the spirit to provide you with healing and restoration. Love, joy, peace, patience, kindness, goodness, faithfulness, gentleness, and self-control are like seeds that when planted, will bloom and flourish into an amazing and abundant harvest of goodness and recovery. These fruits take time and care to grow, but when they come to fruition, you will see that the time and effort were definitely worth it. It is hard to imagine what recovery is like until you are living in it, so hang on to hope and trust me when I say that it is worth it.

I pray that if you are struggling with an ED, this book has inspired you to pursue recovery. Or, if you have already begun, I pray that this equips you with new weapons to fight your battles. Because that is exactly what this is: a battle. The war will be really difficult sometimes, but God will be with you through it all.

Stay strong in your faith, hang on to hope, and don't lose sight of what is truly important. You CAN do this. I believe in you, and I'll be praying for you.

Additional Helpful Tips and Tricks

Coping Cards and Acronyms

Coping cards are a great way to remind yourself of goals or skills to help keep you on track with recovery. All you have to do to make one is write down helpful recovery-focused notes or sayings on an index card or another format of your choosing so that you can easily access it and use it when you need it most. One great thing to include on your coping cards is acronyms that touch on something relevant to you and your recovery. This is a fun activity that I would definitely recommend. Acronyms are especially beneficial because they are easy to remember even when you do not have access to your coping cards. Even if you cannot come up with acronyms, it is still very beneficial to write down your goals or any other mantra or verse on a card to help motivate you. Keep this card with you, and let it help you keep choosing recovery!

Here are some of the acronyms that I have created for myself:

I am
Not
Overcome by the
Ed's
Lies

GOALS:
Go to college
Obtain happiness
Attend to relationships
Live!
Satisfy my purpose in life

BEAUTY is
Being
Enthusiastically
Authentically
Unapologetically
Totally
You!

The Ten Agreements

I have created for myself ten agreements (inspired by the Ten Commandments) that contain a list of commitments that I intend to follow to promote my recovery. You can use mine to inspire your own. Just create for yourself any commitments that you agree to follow that will help keep you on the path of recovery. Make sure that yours is as personalized as it can be. The more meaningful it is to you, the more beneficial it will be.

After you have created your agreements, hang them up in a prominent position that you will frequently see. Mine is on my bedroom door. Then, review these every day and make a daily commitment to live by them. If you slip up, that's okay. Just pick yourself up and get right back on track.

And, if anytime your agreements need to be altered, that's perfectly okay, too. Where people are in their journey is constantly changing, so if needed, update it so that it is the most helpful to you.

It also may be beneficial to share your agreements with your treatment team or support people so that they can help you adhere to them and keep you accountable.

Here's mine to use as a reference or starting point:

The Ten Agreements:

I. I agree to have God be the focus of my life.
The Lord is the One that I will live to serve. In Him, I will put my faith and hope. In Him, I will seek love and acceptance. In Him, I will find meaning and purpose.

II. I agree to no longer follow the eating disorder.
There is only room in my heart for one master, and I choose the Sovereign Lord. As I continue to fight this battle, I agree to trust in God and use my coping strategies. I agree to not let struggles keep me down, but to always get back up and keep fighting.

III. I agree to work on not being so harshly critical of myself, the temple of God.
My approval needs to come from none other than the Lord, and He accepts me for who I am. I will embrace my supposed flaws because they make me unique and help me to grow.

IV. I agree to allow my body to rest.
I will not push myself beyond what I am able, both physically and mentally. I deserve to have rest, and I deserve to give myself time for fun and happiness.

V. I agree to think of my family instead of engaging in the eating disorder.

I love my family far more than I love the eating disorder. The love and acceptance that I crave can all be found from my family: both my loved ones here on earth and from my Heavenly Father.

VI. I agree to not harm my body.
My body does not deserve to be abused or deprived. God gave me this body to take care of, and I agree to love it and nurture it the best that I can.

VII. I agree to be faithful to normalized eating.
Restriction, binging, purging, and other disordered behaviors are not beneficial, and I agree to work on preventing them. If I do begin to slip, I will not allow myself to continue down that spiral. I agree to forgive myself, use my skills, and get back on the right path.

VIII. I agree to no longer allow the eating disorder to steal my life away from me.
God has a purpose and a plan for my life, and I agree to properly nourish my body so that I can live it out. I agree to not allow fears, doubt, or shame keep me from where I want to go: from where I am meant to go.

IX. I agree to not be dishonest.
I will be open and honest with my treatment team, my supports, and with myself. I will be vocal about my struggles and seek help when needed.

X. I agree to accept my body the way that God made it.

God created this body for me and created it good. Even though it may be a long journey, I will continue to practice viewing myself the way that God sees me. He sees me as His beautiful, precious child who has a purpose. He sees me as a temple with Jesus Christ dwelling inside. He calls me loved, worthy, and enough, and that's exactly who I am.

Vision Board

One of the best ways to keep your motivation high and to increase your resilience despite the strongest opposition is to keep in mind your goals and dreams. Knowing what you are working towards helps keep you going. An excellent way to do this is by creating a vision board. You can make a collage, drawing, or write it out. Just use whatever means is most comfortable and meaningful to you.

Make sure that your vision board is as specific and detailed as possible. Allow yourself to fully immerse yourself in the experience and imagine yourself living that life.

Just remember that even though this is your vision, it may not be what God has in store for you. But rest assured in knowing that if that is not what God has planned, He has something even better.

Hang on to dreams, hang on to goals, and hang on to hope. Hope is a powerful thing. God has amazing things planned for you. Keep fighting the good fight.

Here are some questions to get you started on thinking about your vision board:

What do I want to change in my life?
Who do I want to be?
What do I want to do?
How do I want to feel?
Who do I want to be a part of my life?
What would make me happy?
What would give me a sense of purpose and fulfillment?
What do I want my relationship with food to be like?
How do I want to feel about myself?
How would my life be different if I no longer was being held back by the ED?
What would my life look like if I was living for God and not the ED?

About the Author

Noël Deppen is a Christian author who uses her lived experiences to make an impact on the lives of others. For many years, she battled against a fierce eating disorder, but has found freedom once she learned how to turn to God for healing. Now, she is sharing her journey with others to spread the same hope that she has.

www.ingramcontent.com/pod-product-compliance
Lightning Source LLC
LaVergne TN
LVHW041711060526
838201LV00043B/677

Eating disorders (EDs) are devastating illnesses that negatively affect every aspect of one's life. There are many therapies that exist today to challenge ED beliefs, but sufferers often continue to be tormented by the same fears and insecurities. The problem is that even the best treatment is by itself not enough. True healing only comes from the Healer: Jesus Christ.

Feed the Spirit, Starve the ED explores eating disorder recovery through a biblical perspective. By absorbing the fruits of the spirit found in Galatians 5:22-23, individuals can learn how to turn to God for all their needs. Nourishing the soul will fill the void that the ED fails to fill, and it plants the seed for an abundant harvest of life.

For anyone suffering from an eating disorder or those with a loved one in that position, this is the book to read to find healing, freedom, and recovery.